Morning **Yoga** *Workouts*

Zack Kurland

Human Kinetics

Library of Congress Cataloging-in-Publication Data

Kurland, Zack, 1972-
   Morning yoga workouts / Zack Kurland.
      p. cm.
   Includes index.
   ISBN-13: 978-0-7360-6401-9 (soft cover)
   ISBN-10: 0-7360-6401-X (soft cover)
   1. Hatha yoga. 2. Physical fitness. I. Title.
   RA781.7.K87 20007
   613.7'046--dc22

                                            2006023708

ISBN-10: 0-7360-6401-X
ISBN-13: 978-0-7360-6401-9

Acquisitions Editor: Martin Barnard; **Developmental Editor:** Amanda M. Eastin; **Assistant Editors:** Christine Horger and Scott Hawkins; **Copyeditor:** Kathy Calder; **Proofreader:** Anne Rogers; **Indexer:** Betty Frizzéll; **Permission Manager:** Carly Breeding; **Graphic Designer:** Bob Reuther; **Graphic Artist:** Sandra Meier; **Photo Managers:** Joe Jovanovich and Laura Fitch; **Cover Designer:** Keith Blomberg; **Photographer (cover):** K. Vey/Jump; **Photographer (interior):** Thibaut Fagonde; **Art Manager:** Kelly Hendren; **Illustrator:** Concept by Nora and Ted Czukor; redrawn by Kareema McLendon-Foster; **Printer:** United Graphics

Human Kinetics books are available at special discounts for bulk purchase. Special editions or book excerpts can also be created to specification. For details, contact the Special Sales Manager at Human Kinetics.

Printed in the United States of America

10   9   8   7   6   5   4   3   2   1

Human Kinetics
Web site: www.HumanKinetics.com

United States: Human Kinetics
P.O. Box 5076
Champaign, IL 61825-5076
800-747-4457
e-mail: humank@hkusa.com

Canada: Human Kinetics
475 Devonshire Road Unit 100
Windsor, ON N8Y 2L5
800-465-7301 (in Canada only)
e-mail: orders@hkcanada.com

Europe: Human Kinetics
107 Bradford Road
Stanningley
Leeds LS28 6AT, United Kingdom
+44 (0) 113 255 5665
e-mail: hk@hkeurope.com

Australia: Human Kinetics
57A Price Avenue
Lower Mitcham, South Australia 5062
08 8372 0999
e-mail: liaw@hkaustralia.com

New Zealand: Human Kinetics
Division of Sports Distributors NZ Ltd.
P.O. Box 300 226 Albany
North Shore City
Auckland
0064 9 448 1207
e-mail: info@humankinetics.co.nz

This book is dedicated to Blossom,
my original morning yoga companion.

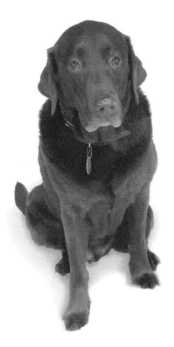

And to my wife, Neena, and our little baby boy, Ravi—
our family, and your love, are the true expression of my yoga.

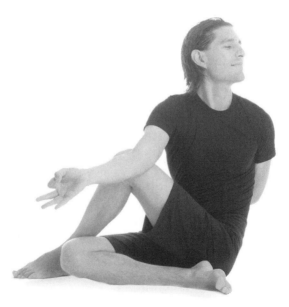

Contents

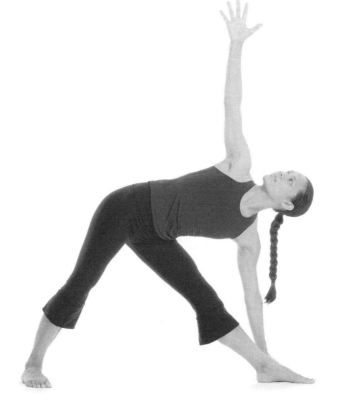

Preface

The day starts the moment you open your eyes. You made the choice to begin your day with a commitment to yoga, health, and happiness. And this book is a tool to help you do that. The idea of yoga as a workout is deeply empowering. Yoga is an ancient system developed over the centuries within the multitude of vedic, tantric, and Buddhist traditions of India and Tibet. These ancient cultures developed the practices of yoga as tools for freedom and self-realization by exploring the nature of the breath, body, mind, and spirit. So why yoga now? How is this ancient esoteric system relevant to getting up and getting fit in modern life?

Your body is your vehicle for exploration, expression, and sensation in this life. Yoga suggests that your level of happiness and freedom is directly influenced by your health. Your state of physical, mental, and emotional well-being directly affects your ability to grow and prosper in every aspect of life. Yoga differs from any other type of exercise in that it encompasses every aspect of well-being. As a workout, yoga will build strength and increase flexibility and stamina. It is well documented that regular yoga practice helps to heal, balance, and optimize digestion, bone density, breath capacity, and endocrine functions. Your physical health and mental and emotional well-being are completely interrelated. The term *workout* not only implies building strength, but it also literally suggests an opportunity to release stress and tension. Through the mindful exercises of yoga, you can actually process the toxicity of stress that accumulates in your body and prevent, or at least minimize, its negative effects on your overall health. The health of your body and mind affects your spirit and quality of life and the way in which you relate with others and your surroundings. Yoga exercise gives you psychical tools as a framework for setting goals, focusing, experiencing accomplishment, and surrendering deeply to develop confidence, understanding, and compassion for yourself and others. In time you will see those qualities manifest in your life off the yoga mat. You may notice a positive shift in the quality of your relationships, your work, and your worldview.

So why practice yoga in the mornings on your own? If you bring the intention of your well-being and self-development to the start of the day, you will most likely have the best chance of succeeding. Intention is not enough! Yoga requires that you take continued action in order to be successful.

When I first started practicing yoga I went to group classes in the afternoon almost every day after work. I was deeply committed. However, afternoons and evenings became more challenging as my responsibilities in work and life grew and changed. I felt "off" on days that I had to miss yoga class and found it difficult to re-create the classes at home. I simply lacked the knowledge and the tools to practice on my own. In time I was fortunate to connect with a teacher who designed a customized yoga practice and encouraged me to practice every morning. With my own yoga practice I could wake up and exercise immediately and reap the benefits of the yoga as I moved forward into the rest of my day. This book simplifies the process by providing a foundation of understanding of yoga and useful tools for the practice of yoga.

Morning time is optimal for yoga practice because you are less likely to let other activities and distractions interfere with your commitment to yoga. Upon waking you have the opportunity to maximize that fresh energy and realize optimal health, happiness, and freedom through yoga.

I offer this book to you as a tool in strengthening your understanding of the principles of breath-centered yoga so that you can immediately begin to develop a robust, enjoyable, and engaging home yoga practice as a means of self-discovery, well-being, and freedom. Regardless of your age, background, or state of health, you can relate to your body and breath. Yoga provides a system for understanding and experiencing your body fully and, in doing so, redefining the boundaries of perceived limitations as you experience new levels of health in your muscles, bones, organs, and tissues. Yoga, in its ancient wisdom, also provides a rich vocabulary and perspective from which you can explore the subtle energies and consciousness that manifest and circulate as life within your body, mind, and spirit. Yoga is not intended as a path to realizing some higher external state. Rather, it is a means of experiencing this life fully with grace and enthusiasm. The linking of breath and movement in yoga exercise reduces physical contraction, energetic obstruction, and the misperception that you are somehow inadequate and separate from the universe. As you engage in yoga exercise you become intimate with the life energy, or prana, you receive through the breath that animates the body. When you maximize your ability to receive this prana through the yogic breath and you exercise your body to become strong and limber, your mind becomes sharp yet adaptable, and your spirit feels connected and receptive to the richness of your experiences in life.

Chapter 1, "Body, Breath, and Mindfulness," contains guidelines for getting started. Part of your yoga practice includes creating an environment in which you can sleep restfully and wake mindfully. Chapter 2, "Morning Energy and Readiness," presents simple guidelines on preparing yourself for yoga exercise and determining what and when to eat and drink to enhance the benefits of your morning yoga workout. You will also explore how to create a physical environment conducive to your yoga practice and address lifestyle factors and responsibilities such as family and pets.

A foundation of understanding yogic breathing, movement, basic anatomy, postural alignment, and subtler energies, applied to your own practical lifestyle considerations, empowers you to move into the physical yoga practices presented in this book, starting with the sun salutations in chapter 3, "Yoga Warm-Ups." Through the sun salutations you become active in experiencing the abundantly bright energy of the sun as your own. By engaging in sun salutations at the start of the day, at the start of yoga practice, you are inherently connected with the power of the sun and the environment by warming up your body and brightening your spirit.

You are then prepared to move deeper into your workout and experience a variety of yoga asanas, or postures, within a series of vinyasas, or sequences, organized within the book by level of intensity: light (chapter 4), moderate (chapter 5), and intense (chapter 6). Each chapter and level of practice has three sequences organized by length of time: 15 to 20 minutes, 30 to 40 minutes, and 50 to 60 minutes, respectively. In this way you can fit your yoga practice into the time available to you without sacrificing the ability to practice yoga regularly. The sequences in chapters 4 through 6 build on one another through the gradual addition and intensification of the exercises so that you can choose an appropriate sequence for you and make progress at your own pace with your available time. Using the three levels of intensity, you can explore yoga within your current ability. The longer morning yoga workouts include specific pranayama, or yogic breathing techniques, for a more refined quality of the breath and aspect of the mind. Through this mindful participation of your breath in pranayama, you tap into the currents of energy moving through your body and are truly present to the wonder of life in the moment. As an expression of this life current in yourself, you can enhance your yoga practice with the use of sound, mantras, creative visualizations, and simple meditations presented in chapter 7, "Visualization and Meditation."

An abundance of traditions and methods make up this vast sea of yoga. Through teachers and personal inclination you may feel more connected to one lineage, style, or tradition than another. I choose to focus on the collective similarities and gifts of all the various yoga lineages and traditions. The paths are many, and each style of yoga or tradition offers its strengths, which make up the diversity that is the spice of life. If at times the information presented in this book conflicts with what you have been taught, I ask only that you commit yourself to your own experience and keep an open mind to determine and find your inner truth.

Acknowledgments

First I'd like to thank and acknowledge my wife, Neena, for her support, encouragement, and patience. She sacrificed all of our weekends while carrying our baby boy, Ravi, so that I could write. I am nothing without your loving belief in me.

I'd like to thank my mother for taking me to my first magical yoga class when I was just 9 years old and then bringing me back to yoga again 15 years later. I owe special thanks to the Kurland and Kumar families for love and life. I offer my deep gratitude to Mohinder, Kanta Devi, and the Sharmas for opening their hearts and sharing their home in the true spirit of India. I also thank Revi for sharing his light, a few ancient Ayurvedic secrets, through his healing hands.

I'd like to acknowledge and thank all of my wonderful, incredible yoga students and clients. You have given me the incredible privilege of living my dream of sharing my love for and belief in yoga.

Thanks go to Mandy Eastin, my editor; Bob Tabian, my literary agent; Martin Barnard; and the staff at Human Kinetics for believing in me enough to realize the vision of this project. Thibaut and Jessica Fagonde expressed their love of yoga through their photography in this book. Steve Rooney and Kathy and Olof Wahlund provided boundless generosity as well as studio space for the photo shoots. Melissa Forbes contributed her beautiful Yantra painting. Kerry Brown and Lululemon Athletica provided beautiful clothing and made me feel like a rock star! Stephanie Creaturo, Blossom Lielani, and Paula Tursi brought the yoga practices within this book to life. I thank all of them for their contributions.

Thanks go to Liz Dreyer, Noah Hilsenrad, and the staff at Learning Worlds for building my wonderful Web site. Thank you to all of the teachers at the Breathing Project for their dedication to sharing and teaching yoga. I thank Mark Whitwell for being an authentic teacher and a true friend, and Cyndi Lee, and the staff and teachers at OM Yoga for their community and support in bringing the teachings of yoga to life every day. Special thanks to Michele Band, Ooi Thye Chong, Matt and Renee Goldman, Gordon McCormick, Gail Papp, Ron Rosbruch, Valerie Smaldone, and Alan Sturm for your support and encouragement. Thank you to T.K.V. and Kausthub Desikachar for generously sharing the yoga teachings of T. Krishnamacharya with the world.

1

Body, Breath, and Mindfulness

The sun is the source of all life; it feeds us and all living beings with vital energy. We awake for a new day with the rising sun. Its energy is our own, and through morning yoga we can link ourselves to its infinite qualities of warmth and illumination. Through our breath and body we can experience the energy of the morning sun in our skin, muscles, and bones. The ancient yogis believed that morning is the most auspicious time for yoga because it is when we are most capable of fully receiving power from the sun and nature. Therefore people through the ages have continued the tradition and covet the practice of yoga in the morning.

The simple practice of engaging our own breath and body through mindfulness is the means by which we fully tap into the power of our connection to the morning sun. In this spirit we come to tangibly experience our breath as the bridge between ourselves and the external environment; we experience our bodies as the living manifestation of the universe itself. But to truly partake of the benefits of morning yoga we must have a concrete means to progress with conscious awareness. In the next chapter you will learn simple practices intended to provide you with tools for incrementally building your yoga practice on a foundation of understanding and adaptability. You must learn how to explore and refine the quality of the breath through specific yogic breathing techniques, while also understanding the classic yogic philosophy behind doing so. This foundation will allow you to engage the body in yoga asanas (exercises and poses) and vinyasas (sequencings of poses), using the breath as the guide to start your morning yoga ritual, and to progress in daily practice with a sense of satisfaction and empowerment.

Breath As the Teacher

In yoga we say, "The breath is life." It is of the utmost importance and truly is the foundation of yoga practice. By focusing on the breath it's possible for each of us to successfully and fully experience yoga, regardless of our age or health. The profound nature of breath animates all living things and links them to one another and to the environment. By exploring the breath within ourselves we connect to the hidden truths within. The breath, being as vast as the ocean, can take us beyond the limitations of self and allow us to grow in new ways through yoga.

In yoga asanas, if we focus on the standard physical forms alone we quickly face limitations through an externally imposed sense of can or can't, bad or good, better or worse. Having the breath as the foundation of yoga practice makes the benefits of yoga available to anyone, through its commonality and expansive nature, without imposing a standardized approach to the asanas and physical forms associated with yoga. The breath both allows us to experience yoga postures deeply and tells us when to back off and take rest. Through the breath we can cultivate a quiet mind by simply noticing the rhythmic rising and falling of our chest. Connecting the yoga postures and movements to the breath ensures safe practice, prevents injury, and maximizes the therapeutic benefit of yoga practice. Unfolding the movements within a posture and enveloping the transitions within the breath itself adds fluidity and helps us avoid forcing ourselves into postures prematurely.

For years I have experienced steady growth and continually expanding boundaries in my personal yoga practice and with countless students. Through breathing, an opening process occurs on the structural, muscular, and energetic planes. Surrendering to the exhalation releases any resistance in the muscles so that we can fully receive the invigorating energy of the morning through our inhalation. Through breath-centered yoga we go deeper, gradually becoming more open and accepting.

This next section outlines two breathing exercises that lay a solid foundation for yogic breathing. They will enable you to attend first to the quality of the breath and then to the breath's relationship with the body in some of the simplest movements associated with yoga asanas. The breathing techniques presented here help you to develop a robust way of breathing that we will build on throughout the book as you progress in practice. Although there is no correct way to breathe, we can certainly work toward optimizing our use of the breath by being mindful of its quality and length and then establishing specific yogic breathing methods that enhance our experience in the physical exercises.

Breathing for Interconnectivity

This breathing exercise is the first step toward developing our yogic breath through a progression of techniques. With this technique we can begin to experience on a cellular level what the ancient teachings known as the Yoga Sutra of Patanjali call the *union of yoga*. By concentrating pointedly on the breath, we experience the union between the breath and ourselves. The more frenetic frequencies of the mind dissipate, allowing us to more clearly understand the true nature of that which we are observing as ourselves. Recognizing the interconnectivity, let's try a simple yogic meditation exercise to consciously experience the union of breath and body as part of a larger progression of exercises.

1. Lie on the back. Close the eyes and relax. Observe the natural breath rising and falling.
2. Begin to lengthen the inhalation and deepen the exhalation.
3. Explore the boundaries of the inhalation and the depths of the exhalation without struggle or strain for 6 breaths.
4. Add a slight pause between the inhalation and exhalation to create a four-part breath: Inhale, pause in; exhale, pause out. Continue with this long, smooth, four-part breathing for 12 breaths.
5. Release the pauses between inhalation and exhalation, letting the long inhalation flow into deep exhalation for 6 more breaths.
6. Let go of the breath completely and just observe the natural breath rising and falling again, free of effort. Be mindful of how you feel during this simple yet profound practice.

This exercise is a wonderful way to experience the breath in four parts and discover your breath capacity. In doing so you may have cultivated a different state of mind. Each part of the breath has unique qualities. We receive the breath and thus draw in energy from our environment. Holding the breath in, we can fully absorb this energy. Through the exhalation we assert our strength and at the same time release from within what we no longer need. Holding the breath out after the exhalation, we can relax into the emptiness and soften. In this way we can tangibly experience the breath on the physical, mental, and emotional levels. Let go of any judgments about your breath quality or capacity. Allow it to act as a vehicle of change as you progress in yoga practice.

Now that you have learned to concentrate on the breath and consciously experience it, you must next learn how the breath and body work together in movement. In this next exercise we will learn to bring consciousness to the movements of the body in relation to the breath—the next step in our development of yoga as the seamless union of breath, body, and mindfulness. Later, within the practice portion of the book, we will more clearly examine the dynamics of the specific asanas themselves, within the appropriate sequences designed to maximize the benefit of your morning yoga workouts.

The ancient yogic texts describe the asanas as physical postures that can be sustained with a balance of stability (*sthira*) and ease (*sukha*). Through yoga practice we learn to establish such stability and ease within the postures through the breath, using the breathing techniques we just learned as well as those presented later in the chapter. This morning yoga of breath, body, and mindfulness maintains the interplay between stability and ease, or strength and receptivity, through breath. By doing so at the start of our day on a regular basis we will experience these qualities of strength, stability, receptivity, and ease in our physical, mental, emotional, and spiritual being throughout the rest of the day.

I believe that the body can reflect the nature of breath. Our aim is to cultivate long and steady breath without strain. By placing the movements within the breath length itself, we will establish a direct relationship in which we can easily maintain that balance of stability and ease. When our yoga asana is too rigid or strained we may find our breath short or restricted, or we may notice that we are not breathing at all. If we are too rigid in breath or movement we run the risk of strain and injury. In this state we inhibit our ability to be receptive and impinge on the energy flow throughout our system. Likewise, when we are not alert our yoga asana will be sluggish and our breathing shallow. If the breath or muscular quality of the body is too soft or mushy, then we lack the strength to move forward and sustain a given direction. In yoga practice we aim to establish and maintain a balance of opposite but complementary qualities. As we progress, we see how the qualities of stability and suppleness are manifest not only in our yoga asana exercises but also in our state of mind on and off the yoga mat.

Let's try another simple awareness exercise, building on the first, to bring mindfulness to the unity of breath and body. By consciously enveloping the movements within the breath itself, the body can reflect the stability and ease of the breath.

1. Lie on the back with the arms alongside the body. (See figure 1.1*a*.)
2. As before, begin to lengthen the breath, extending inhalation and deepening exhalation to your breath capacity.
3. Add a slight pause between inhalation and exhalation to establish a four-part breath.
4. Start the next inhalation and begin the movement a second later, lifting the arms back overhead in line with the body. (See figure 1.1*b*.)
5. Start the next exhalation and begin the movement a second later, bringing the arms back down along the sides in line with the body.
6. Continue for 6 breaths, consciously starting the movement slightly after the start of the breath.
7. As you continue, try to make the breath longer than the movement. Finish the breath a second or two after you finish the arm movements, both on inhalation and exhalation (you may find you need to adjust the pace of the movements). This practice creates a full breath envelope. Continue for another 10 breaths.

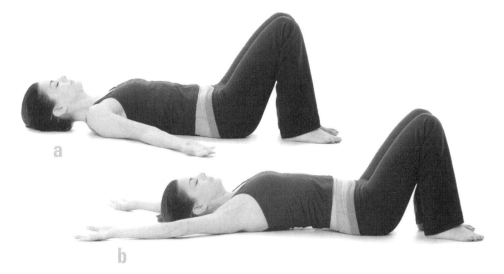

FIGURE 1.1   Breathing awareness exercise: *(a)* arms alongside the body; *(b)* arms overhead in line with the body.

We have created a framework in which the movements of the body directly relate to both the quality and length of the breath. Later in this chapter we will discuss additional simple breathing methods that allow you to increase the quality and length of the breath without strain.

The breathing awareness exercises we have just completed give us the tools to build this foundation of stability and ease. One of my yoga teachers often said, "You can bully the body, but you can't cheat the breath." We can maintain a conscious awareness of breath quality that is long, smooth, and steady, transferring these qualities to the body during movement and stillness.

When practicing a yoga asana we will often do several repetitive or dynamic movements before maintaining a static posture. This dynamic movement establishes the breath-to-body relationship and prepares us for the full expression of a static yoga asana. In this way we can flow through the vinyasas and maintain postures without strain or injury. If we come into yoga postures cold, we may experience rigidity or resistance. By using dynamic movements to prepare for held postures, we can maintain the breath-to-body link to give our yoga a more profound layer of depth. Now that we know how to coordinate the breath and the movements of the body, the next step is to learn how to coordinate our yogic breathing with the abdominal musculature in order to promote strength and stability.

Breathing for Improved Energy and Digestion

One of the benefits of morning yoga is that through yogic breath and physical exercises we can truly affect the amount of energy we have at the start of our day. The ancient techniques described in this book have real value in our fast-paced lives. By breathing deeply and engaging the body through moving and held postures, we will eliminate sluggishness and make the morning a special time for the personal ritual of practice, bringing a renewed sense of pleasure and anticipation to our waking.

Yoga is fun to do—it feels great and keeps us animated and attentive throughout the day. This energy is what the yogis called *prana*. It is the energy that flows throughout our system and animates us. The yogis described prana as the life-sustaining energy we receive through the breath and food. I also believe that we receive prana from all of our surroundings, including our personal relationships and what we see and hear. This is the life essence, called *rasa* or juice of life, and it is necessary for health and happiness.

For now let's focus how we receive prana through air and food. Prana's primary location is the lungs and respiratory system. Our body receives prana through breath and food and then distributes it by means of the circulatory system. In yoga our aim is to maximize our ability to receive prana and distribute it throughout the body as effectively and efficiently as possible. Both the air and the food we ingest create waste, which needs to be released from the body. In yoga this force of elimination is called *apana*.

Through aging, lifestyle, habits, and accumulated tension we may develop physical, mental, emotional, and spiritual obstacles or blocks in our system. The yogis perceived a major contributing factor to the blocks to be an accumulation of waste in the apana region of the body, which is located primarily around the lower abdomen. The breathing and physical exercises of yoga provide us with incredible methods to help release accumulated waste, toxins, and stress so that we experience good health and effectively receive, distribute, and assimilate the prana from our air and food. In this way we experience the benefits of yoga physically, mentally, and emotionally through increased breath capacity and improved digestion, assimilation, and elimination.

The yogis believed that we can maintain or regain good health through a strong metabolic and digestive ability. They thought of this digestive ability as an internal fire called *agni*. This agni resides mainly in the midsection of the torso at the location of the stomach, liver, pancreas, and gall bladder, all of which contain acid and bile and are responsible for breaking down and processing food and toxins. The digestive fire, agni, diminishes over time through the accumulation of excess waste in the apana region. The force of apana is downward in the direction of elimination, except for the breath, which leaves the body by moving upward through exhalation. Engaging the musculature of the lower abdomen during exhalation moves the accumulation of waste in the apana region toward the midsection, where agni resides. The yogis believed this excess is burned off through our internal combustion, thereby fanning our internal fire through breath and increasing the strength of agni over time. As the accumulation of waste in the lower abdomen dissipates, our digestive fire increases so that we can more effectively eliminate waste and absorb prana from our food. Practicing yoga in the morning is extremely effective for releasing the accumulated waste and toxins of the previous day so that you can start the new day fresh and clear, fully prepared to receive new food and energy.

Attention to the use of abdominal musculature during exhalation also results in increased strength and stability in the lower torso. As a result, the muscles of the upper torso and back need to work less and can relax, giving us increased mobility and breathing capacity so that we can more effectively receive our prana through the breath. Let's do another exercise to experience how we can increase the use of the lower abdominal musculature, reduce toxins, and improve metabolism and digestion through yogic breathing.

1. Lie on the back. Place one hand on the upper chest and the other on the lower abdomen, right below the navel. (See figure 1.2.) Breathe freely, observing the rising and falling of the chest.

2. Initiate and deepen the exhalation at the lower abdomen by drawing the belly in toward the spine and up toward the ribs, drawing the hand in and up. Finish the exhalation with the hand on the upper chest falling last.

3. Initiate and lengthen the inhalation through an expansion of breath as the ribs, upper torso, and top hand lift. As the expansion through the chest continues, notice that the pressure moves downward toward the belly and that the lower hand lifts as a result.

4. Place a slight pause between the inhalation and the exhalation, as we did in the earlier exercise, and repeat for about 10 breaths.

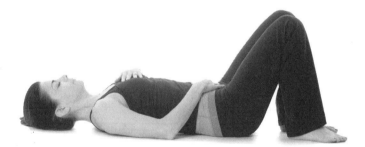

FIGURE 1.2   Hand position on upper chest and lower abdomen.

This type of breathing may differ from other yogic techniques frequently taught. It has the specific purpose of engaging the musculature of the lower torso on the exhalation to increase strength and stability and to draw the apana region toward the midsection, where the agni resides. Also, the muscular actions associated with breathing occur naturally and can result in the benefits of improved digestion, assimilation, increased breath capacity, elimination of waste, and abdominal and spinal support.

Ujjayi: Ocean Breathing

We have learned to bring awareness and intention to yogic breathing. Now we are ready to learn how to breathe robustly in the more complex yogic exercises and poses presented later in this book. The yogic breathing techniques we are going to learn now use ujjayi, or ocean breathing, to regulate the breath during a yoga asana; it is also an adjunct pranayama practice in itself, either before or after yoga asanas. *Pranayama* means to extend the life force, through the extension of the breath capacity. Ujjayi breathing provides us with a method to refine the quality and length of the breath and to enhance all of the aspects of yoga practice we have discussed. Ujjayi is often called ocean breathing and sounds like waves drawing in and out on the shore. You can experience it by slightly contracting the larynx or vocal chords so that there is a soft constriction at the throat. When you do ujjayi correctly, the breath will make this foggy ocean sound. This method enables us to monitor the breath quality through sound and to pace the rate of inhalation and exhalation by limiting the size of the air passage. By means of the stabilizing use of musculature in the upper torso, ujjayi provides us with an additional and necessary support during yoga asanas. It is generally easier to learn ujjayi breathing on exhalation, but in time you should apply it during inhalation as well. Let's try a simple exercise so that you can experience it for yourself.

1. Take a comfortable seated or lying position. Inhale freely.

2. Open the mouth like you are going to fog up or clean a pair of glasses. Contract the throat ever so slightly and exhale through the mouth, making a foggy ocean sound. If this is confusing, try saying "ha" out loud to engage the contraction of the vocal chords and then release the vocalization while retaining the contraction. Try it a few times, playing with the contraction at the throat and the shape of the mouth until you can make the sound.

3. Once you can establish and maintain the contraction at the throat, try to make the same foggy noise on inhalation while breathing through the mouth. If this seems difficult, don't be discouraged—it will come with practice. Continue breathing through the mouth, relaxing any unnecessary tension so that the breath is smooth and steady on both inhalation and exhalation.

4. Close the mouth and try to make the same foggy noise at the throat while breathing through the nose. Switch back and forth until you begin to get the hang of it.

Learning ujjayi breathing is often challenging at first, but in time it will feel like second nature. I cannot overstate the profound depth that ujjayi breathing adds to yoga practice. Some would argue that without ujjayi, breathing while doing asanas and vinyasas is not yoga. The ujjayi inhalation is often the key to full receptivity of prana. Continued practice of ujjayi will allow us to increase mobility and breath length without straining the neck and shoulders. In addition, this ujjayi, or ocean breathing, gives us a focal point on which to fix our concentration, bringing about a meditative peace of mind. Become aware of its presence throughout your yoga practice each morning and continually draw your concentration back to ujjayi breathing when the mind begins to wander. Notice how you can monitor postural alignment in yoga asanas with the aid of ujjayi breathing. Overexertion, tension, or sluggishness will surely be reflected in the waves of the breath. I suggest you try all of the exercises presented thus far again using ujjayi breathing, and notice how it increases your ability to concentrate and to experience the relationship of breath, body, and mind.

We can also do ujjayi pranayama as an adjunct practice, either before or after we finish our yoga asanas. In this way we minimize our focus on the body during yoga pranayama and explore the breath's more subtle qualities in a fixed position. A multitude of possibilities exists for using ujjayi pranayama to cultivate calm, focus energy, and promote mental clarity. To experience the benefits, we can practice ujjayi pranayama sitting or lying, breathing freely or with breath counts; we can also use bandha (discussed later in this chapter) for varying degrees of intensity. I will outline specific practices to complement your morning yoga asanas, but use your sense of intuition to explore the boundaries of the breath and of the internal landscape of the breath capacity and its relationship to body, mind, and spirit that can be revealed through ujjayi pranayama.

Nadi Sodhana: Alternate Nostril Breathing

Another pranayama that is useful for balance, clarity, and peace of mind is nadi sodhana, or alternate nostril breathing. You should do this pranayama (unlike ujjayi) only in a seated position on the floor or in a chair, either before or after yoga asanas, because you must maintain a straight spine throughout, and you must use the hand in what is called a *mudra*, or hand gesture, to regulate the use of the nostrils. The yogis believed that this pranayama could balance the polarities between left and right, male and female, hot and cold, represented within the nadis *ida* and *pingala* that run alongside the spine.

1. Take a comfortable seated position. Extend the right hand forward with the palm facing up. Bring the index and middle fingers into the palm (see figure 1.3*a*).

2. Bring the right hand to the nose, placing the ring finger on the left nostril and the thumb on the right, just below the bridge bone.

3. To begin, take one full breath, inhaling and exhaling through both nostrils.

4. Close off the left nostril completely with the ring finger and inhale through the right (see figure 1.3*b*). Hold the breath in, using the ring finger and the thumb to close both nostrils; lower the chin toward the chest. Release the ring finger and exhale through the left nostril. Hold the breath out for a few seconds.

5. Inhale through the left nostril. Close both nostrils and hold the breath in for a few seconds. Release the right nostril and exhale. This completes one full round of alternate nostril breathing. Throughout the breathing exercise, the chin should rise away from the chest naturally to take and release breath and remain toward the chest during the pauses between.

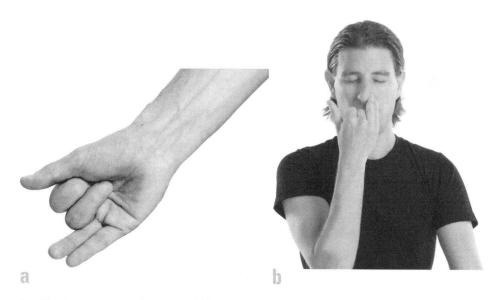

FIGURE 1.3   Alternate nostril breathing: *(a)* finger position, *(b)* hand position.

6. Repeat this cycle for six full rounds or 12 breaths, finishing with an exhalation through the right nostril.
7. Relax the hand down, breathe freely, and observe how you feel.

Body Consciousness

We have learned the importance of breath and of its relation to the body through mindfulness. Yoga as a form of exercise allows us to develop ourselves throughout a full spectrum of levels—physically, mentally, emotionally, and spiritually. Although other types of exercise may focus on more than one area, I can think of no other form of exercise that addresses our whole being so completely. For this reason millions of people use the many gifts of yoga to reconnect, develop, and transform themselves. The exercises and poses in yoga (asanas) and the sequencing of poses (vinyasas) are a wonderful way to engage the body through consciousness so that we can build strength and flexibility through building lean, toned muscle mass. Through yoga asanas and vinyasas we can increase structural mobility by bringing the spine, torso, and limbs through their full range of movement to keep the body fluid (juicy with synovial fluid). We do so with attention to postural alignment so that we don't compromise the integrity of the joints, ligaments, cartilage, and connective tissue. Morning yoga workouts will increase balance and improve core stability through directed muscular engagement and will preserve bone strength through weight-bearing exercise. The morning ritual of yoga will cultivate increased stamina and endurance. Moving through the poses and sequences with fluidity will bring increased coordination. By embodying the asanas themselves with an enlightened awareness, you will feel physically energized and mentally and emotionally grounded.

As human beings we all share the same basic anatomy and physiology. But we are also unique individuals—each of us is different in size, shape, character, and constitution. Therefore each of us requires an individualized approach to yoga. But we don't have to reinvent the wheel with each person. Most likely, all of us will practice some variation of the same yoga postures and perhaps even a similar sequence. The sequences presented within this book are very effective tools for starting your own yoga practice each morning.

Yoga Asanas

The asanas, or physical postures, associated with yoga practice are the main focus of our morning workouts and serve as a framework for our experience and transformation. Within these forms we can explore how to cultivate the manifestation of breath and energy in the muscles, bones, organs, and tissues of our bodies. The ancient yogis discovered that by emulating the shapes of the animals and forms that exist in nature they could maintain good health, develop the physical body, and expand consciousness. We discussed earlier that the asanas must maintain a balance of supportive strength and comfortable ease. It's easy to get caught up in the physical forms themselves and strive to achieve the obscure asanas we have seen in books, in videos, and even at yoga classes. Instead, we must respect our present state, the current needs of our body, and the messages of the breath. You can injure yourself doing complicated asanas as contortions or exotic gymnastics. I speak from personal experience; I have injured myself through wrong practice, to the point of needing knee surgery. So I encourage students to practice yoga asanas in relation to the breath and through primary spinal orientation (discussed in the next section).

The asanas fall into several basic categories, based on their spinal orientation. These asanas are presented according to their classifications on pages 211-212. Within these classifications, you can do asanas while standing, seated, lying face up (supine), lying face down (prone), or upside down. Some asanas, like pincha mayurasana (forearm stand), which is both an inversion and a deep backbend, fall within multiple categories.

The sequencing of postures, or how we flow from asana to asana, is called *vinyasa krama*. As we discussed earlier, morning yoga practice is energetically more *brmhana*, or energizing, and the vinyasas I present later in the book are meant to wake us up through an increase of activity. As a rule, simple asanas prepare us for more complex ones, gradually moving toward what I call peak asanas, such as urdva danurasana (full wheel) or sirsasana (headstand). You can easily identify these peak asanas as the more challenging poses around which the full yoga practice, or a specific vinyasa, is oriented. Asanas, especially peak asanas, take our bodies in a particular direction structurally, muscularly, and energetically. They require counterposing to release any accumulated muscular, structural, and emotional tension so that we finish yoga practice feeling balanced and free of pain. In many cases, counterposing is just good common sense; it may be as simple and intuitive as hugging the knees into the chest, or taking a twist, after deeper back bending. The vinyasas in the book offer sequences of classic asanas and the necessary counterposes, with adaptations to maximize therapeutic efficacy and minimize risk of injury, or to increase intensity so that the yoga is adequately challenging. The best complement for these yoga practices is a personal relationship with a qualified yoga teacher, whose insight and perspective can provide instruction and clarity when there is confusion or doubt.

Yoga and the Spine

We have thus far explored the breathing and energetic vocabularies associated with yoga. The yoga asanas that are generally of most benefit are those that are primarily oriented to the spine. The spine forms the core of our body and houses the central nervous system. The central nervous system emerges from the brain, extends down through the spine, and then branches out to the peripheral extremities of the arms and legs. Movements in yoga practice should engage the spine by facilitating mobility and stability within its full range of directions, without bullying or straining it beyond its capacity. We use the breath as a means to gauge the quality, intensity, and duration of our yoga asana practice.

The spine runs from the base of the skull down to the end of the tailbone. The central nervous system emerges from the brain stem, and it is housed within the vertebrae. It branches outward into a network of intelligence throughout the body. Much of the major musculature is anchored to the spine. The internal organ systems that are housed with the muscular and skeletal systems are oriented along the spine as well. The spine and breath have a significant relationship because of the insertion of the diaphragm and ribs at the spine. The unique curvature and vertebral configuration within human beings has developed over millions of years to allow us to stand, alone in nature. The spine is both stable and flexible. We find the many keys to opening up to a deep, successful, and satisfying yoga practice when we orient the yoga asanas and vinyasas around spinal movement. We should explore the spine's full range of movement and experience the stability and mobility of the shoulders, hips, legs, and arms emerging as a peripheral extension of spinal orientation.

The spine is made up of several sections. The neck contains 7 cervical vertebrae, and 12 thoracic vertebrae form the upper back and midsection. The lumbar spine has 5 vertebrae, and the sacrum has 5 more. The structure of the vertebrae changes to allow for more mobility at the top of the spine and more stability at the base. Collectively, the vertebrae form four major curves along the vertical plane. The first curve at the cervical spine is known as lordosis, the second at the thoracic spine is kyphosis, the third is lordosis again at the lumbar spine, and the fourth is a kyphotic inward curve at the sacral spine. These curves exist naturally to varying degrees within each of us. Through regular yoga practice we can help minimize and possibly correct imbalances such as a collapsed chest or humped back, often indicative of tension, stress, or a lack of structural integrity common in women and men with osteopenia and osteoporosis. In addition, it is natural and fairly common for there to be curvatures along the horizontal plane of the spine to varying degrees. More extreme cases, as seen in scoliosis, usually have some component of rotational irregularity and may cause discomfort. Yoga can help regulate these tendencies, minimize pain, and inhibit further negative developments, even in individuals in whom the spine has a very unique expression.

In yoga we take the spine through an array of movements. Let's explore these a bit.

- **Flexion** occurs when the front of the spine shortens. It is associated with forward bending movements during exhalation in yoga asanas.
- **Extension** occurs when the back of the spine shortens. It is associated with backward bending movements during inhalation in yoga asanas.
- **Rotation** occurs when the spine twists along the axial plane. It is associated with twisting movements during exhalation in yoga asanas.
- **Lateral flexion** occurs when one side of the spine lengthens. It is associated with side bending movements on both inhalation and exhalation in yoga asanas.

All of the poses and movements in yoga asanas take the spine into one of these four types of movement, or some combination of them. Remember that we can injure the spine when pushing ourselves beyond its capabilities. So I often find myself instructing, "Breathe, don't bully, the spine." Because of internal changes in both volume and pressure during breathing, the spine requires increased space during inhalation to allow for expansion of the ribs and thoracic cavity. We can also deepen the poses and movements of the spine as we engage the exhalation. Extension of the spine in backward bending is more associated with inhalation, whereas forward bends and twists are more associated with exhalation. We engage the spine in rotation on exhalation, whereas inhalation requires us to back off slightly and soften the asana for the breath. We usually perform side bends on exhalation, but we can experience expansion during the inhalation through the long side of the body on a side bend. These four types of movement allow us to experience the full intelligence of the spine in relation to the profound nature of the breath and the supportive musculature at the body's core.

Core Stability

By engaging the strength of the lower body through exhalation, we establish our first connection to the core stability so often talked about in yoga and Pilates. In yoga we establish this core stability through breathing and engaging the muscles at three energetic locks called *bandhas*. The first is *mula bandha*, or root lock, which we engage when we initiate the exhalation at the base of the body, using the pelvic floor and the lower abdominal muscles. Over time we will develop this connection and strengthen our base support. We can choose to release mula bandha prior to inhalation, as we have in the earlier breathing exercises, or to keep engaging it throughout the following inhalation. The second bandha is *udayana bandha*, or flying upward lock, and we establish it at the diaphragm and upper abdominal muscles. This bandha occurs naturally as we deepen the exhalation and engage the upper abdominal muscles and the musculature of the middle torso. We can experience the full expression of udayana bandha during the pause after exhalation by scooping the belly in and up under the ribs while holding the breath out. We engage the third bandha, *jalandhara bandha* or throat lock, when we seal the air passageway to hold the breath in or out. We can also employ it by lengthening the back of the neck and lowering the chin toward the chest, while still allowing for controlled breathing.

All three bandhas collectively make up core stability. They are interrelated by their orientation around the breath and the musculature of the torso. By bringing awareness and intention to our quality of breath and energy in relation to the body during yoga practice, we can experience a less rigid application of bandha energetically, structurally, and muscularly. The bandhas are fully integrated and are a natural occurrence of the yogic breathing process, rather than a separate muscular action that we impose on ourselves.

Let's try another exercise to experience accessing the core support of yogic bandha through muscular engagement and breath.

1. Lie on the back. Bend the knees and bring the feet to the floor about hip-width apart (see figure 1.4*a*).

2. Inhale, filling the chest, and then let the pressure expand to the lower abdomen. Hold the breath in. Here we experience jalandhara bandha on the pause after inhalation.

3. Relax the throat. Start the exhalation by engaging mula bandha through the muscles of the lower abdomen. As you continue to exhale, let the chest drop. Hold the breath out. Maintain mula bandha by keeping the muscles of the lower belly drawn in.

4. Release jalandhara bandha at the throat. Inhale, take the arms back overhead in line with the body, and lift the hips (see figure 1.4*b*). Keep the hips lifted and exhale fully, engaging mula bandha by drawing the belly in throughout the breath.

5. Close the throat, engaging jalandhara bandha. Hold the breath out and lower the hips, while keeping the arms back behind you (see figure 1.4*c*). Notice any suction you may feel at the midsection or diaphragm—this is udayana bandha.

6. Relax the throat and inhale.

7. Repeat the exercise 10 times and see whether you can experience the three bandhas through simple breath and movement.

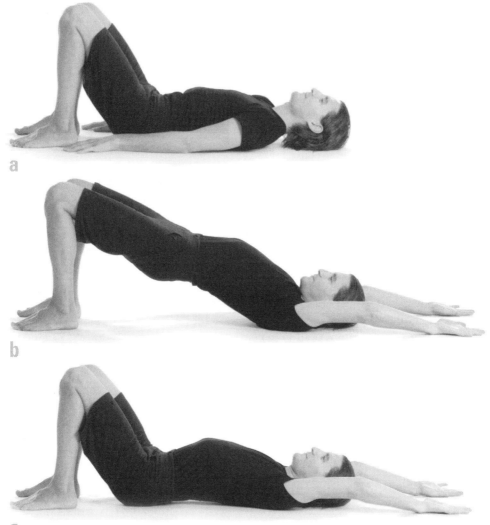

FIGURE 1.4   Bandha exercise: *(a)* lying on back; *(b)* hips lifted and arms overhead; *(c)* hips lowered.

A direct connection exists between using bandha, or core stability, and improving digestion and elimination. The ancient yogis, developing their language for mapping the processes of gross and subtle bodies, believed that through the use of bandha, the yogi could draw the lower abdominal area, which is the seat of the apana region, in and up toward the midsection, the seat of agni. As the pelvic floor lifts in mula bandha and as the upper abdominal muscles and diaphragm lift upward in udayana bandha, the energetic and physical obstacles of the lower abdomen can be reduced by our own internal heat.

These bandhas occur naturally as an extension of the breath, and by placing them intentionally throughout yoga practice we can increase strength, stability, and mental focus. Over time the consistent use of the abdominal muscles in mula and udayana bandha develops our ability to access the core musculature and develop muscular strength. By using breath-based bandha we become experts in assessing proper structural alignment through proper muscular engagement.

Postural Alignment

We must be conscious of postural alignment in yoga asanas. This topic can be confusing, since there are many schools of thought about what determines correct postural alignment. Such confusion is yet another reason for practicing yoga asanas and vinyasas grounded in the breath and spinal orientation. By maintaining the balance of sthiram (stability) and sukham (space) we can be conscious of when and where specific areas of the body feel overstressed or collapsed.

Listen to the messages of the breath and body. If you feel pain, back off or stop and take rest. We can gradually increase muscular flexibility and strength but, as a rule, the soft tissue of the joints should be supported through muscular action, not stressed. Cartilage and ligaments, particularly in the knees and shoulders, have poor blood supply and do not heal easily. Often there is a misperception that you should work through pain or tension. I prefer to listen to the breath and respect current limitations, allowing for gradual progress. There is a tendency to collapse into the joints in yoga asanas for a false sense of stability. You can avoid this inclination by adding a slight bend at the joints, which takes away this unnecessary strain to the soft tissue and allows the musculature of the arms, legs, and feet to engage naturally.

Be mindful of tendencies to let the body's weight fall completely into one leg when practicing standing postures like trikonasana (triangle pose) or to collapse into the shoulders during arm-supported asanas such as urdva mukha svanasana (upward-facing dog). Engage the musculature of the limbs and lift out of the collapsed area, establishing energetic balance in an asana. Also be aware of neck and back tension from overexertion or from extreme spinal flexion, extension, and rotation. We can simplify the technical instructions slightly by making intuitive adjustments and subtle variations to asanas, with the intention of creating space for the inhalation, and then engaging the lower abdominal musculature for core stability during the exhalation. Focusing on the breath allows much of the postural alignment to occur naturally. It should take only a moment or two to set up in any given posture. Then we maintain postural integrity throughout the asana with continued awareness of the relationship between body and breath.

Nadis and Chakras: Subtle Body of Yoga Practice

Union, the very definition of yoga, implies that our aims are to create a conscious awareness of how things relate and to establish a balance between them. In yoga asanas, we bring that awareness and balance into our breath and body through mindfulness and increased strength, stability, flexibility, focus, coordination, and energy. In this way, yoga is a moving meditation and affects the quality of the mind. The ideas and exercises we've covered provide a framework from which our morning yoga practices can emerge.

Each yoga practice has a distinct energetic quality and effect on our systems. We must determine though self-examination how our yoga practices can give us langhana (release and relaxation) or brmhana (energizing and strengthening), or an equal balance of both. Determining what makes a yoga practice more langhana or more brmhana has to do with who you are; with the intensity, types, and sequencing of asanas and breathing exercises; and with the length of a particular yoga practice. Yoga done in the morning is inherently brmhana because of the rising sun and the start of the day. However, our morning yoga practice should be a satisfyingly balanced combination of invigoration and relaxation so that we start the day feeling energized and relaxed, not wiped out or groggy. I have created general practices for a diversity of people to practice yoga in the morning on their own. When using the book you must honor and respect your individuality so that you can choose a yoga practice that truly suits your present needs.

The ancient yogis mapped how they perceived human energy and consciousness within the human system through a complex system of passageways called *nadis* and *chakras*. There are 72,000 nadis, of which three are said to be important and one supreme. This supreme nadi is *susumna*, the central channel that runs along the spine. *Ida* represents female, cooler energy—the moon or *ha*—and starts at the left nostril. *Pingala* represents the male, hotter energy—the sun or *tha*. Together, these two polarities of left and right, female and male, moon and sun, and cold and hot form hatha yoga. These two nadis crisscross along susumna at the seven chakra centers. The chakras are energetic vortexes along the central channel where certain types of energy and consciousness manifest physically within us. They are the following:

- *Muladhara*—Root chakra at the base of the spine. In terms of energy, this area reflects stability, support, and our instinctual need for food, shelter, and survival.

- *Svadhisthana*—The navel or navel region. This area reflects sustenance, reproduction, and relationship.

- *Manipura*—The solar plexus. The seat of agni, this area reflects combustion, digestion, transformation, and ability to adapt to change.

- *Anahata*—The heart chakra. In terms of energy, this area reflects our capacity for openness and connectivity, for giving and receiving love.

- *Vishuddhi*—The throat chakra. This area reflects the ability to communicate and express ourselves.

- *Ajna*—Known as the third eye chakra. This area reflects inherent self-knowledge and deeper perceptive ability to comprehend the universal and interconnected nature of our being.

- *Sahasra*—The crown chakra. This area reflects the ability to transcend our perceived limitations and move toward a more universal understanding of self.

At the base of susumna, at muladhara chakra, is what the yogis called the *kundalini*. My teachers described the kundalini as an obstruction at the base of the spine, where ida and pingala meet and enter susumna. This obstruction is thought to inhibit the full flow of the primary life force, prana, up through susumna. We discussed earlier in this chapter how we can minimize the accumulation of waste in the apana region through the use of our digestive fire and the strength of the exhalation. We can also use the same action of engaging the lower musculature of the abdomen to minimize or eliminate this perceived obstruction of kundalini by drawing it toward the digestive fire, agni, to be burned off. As this process occurs, the prana can flow more freely up through the main channel, susumna.

I prefer to think of the vocabulary of this ancient yoga system as a metaphoric language created to explain the inherent intelligence of the spine and subtle energetic phenomena that occur within the human system, affecting body, breath, mind, and spirit. There are many books that go into the nadi and chakra system in greater detail. For the purposes of morning yoga, it is useful to acknowledge that we exist as energetic beings within the vehicle of our physical body. Within each of us, certain character traits and tendencies are more apparent and dominant than others. If we listen to our body, heart, and mind, we will have sufficient guidance to fully benefit from practicing yoga each morning.

Yoga and Other Physical Activities

The yoga practices presented in this book are perfect as the cornerstone of a personal approach to wellness. Up to this point, we have discussed morning yoga as an activity in itself, to be done prior to going to work or taking care of family responsibilities, since for most this will comprise the majority of our days. However, our morning yoga practice could and should include weekends and leisure time as well. It's no secret, and no surprise, that many world-class athletes, on teams like the New York Jets and in world-class dance companies like the Alvin Ailey American Dance Theater, already incorporate regular yoga practice into their training schedules.

For most of us, the appropriate amount of yoga can provide the perfect warm-up or cool-down before or after other recreational and physical activities. For example, I have a yoga student who loves to play golf. His goal when I first met him was primarily to improve his flexibility. He was concerned that, as the years went by, he had lost a considerable amount of flexibility, and he felt limited in his ability to perform everyday tasks like reaching the floor to pick up a pen or tying his shoes. Like most adult professionals, he spent most of his time at the office behind a desk or in a car going to and from his office and clients. But his true passion was golf. It became clear that his main source of stress relief and a primary source of pleasure was his weekend golf game. I asked him to do a short yoga practice before he left the house to play and to see what happened. After doing so, he was surprised that almost immediately he had an increased range of motion in his upper body and more stability through his legs. He was even more surprised at the benefit of increased mental focus from doing just 20 minutes of yoga before he played golf. He was happy to improve his game with long drives, more accurate putting, and a full experience of the simple pleasure of spending an afternoon with friends outside in the fresh air and sun. This is just one example of how yoga can maximize the pleasure we derive from our recreational activities.

On a given morning, estimate how much time you have for one of the well-rounded yoga practices in this book. Gauge the amount of energy you need to conserve, or have already expended, to choose the appropriate amount of time and level of intensity. It's not useful to do the one-hour intensive practice if you are going to play, or have just played, three hours of tennis. In yoga, maximizing the uninhibited flow of energy, or prana, in our system is the goal—not depleting your energy by overexertion and paying the price by being exhausted or even risking injury. If the physical activity you do for pleasure comes at a physical price, then doing a little yoga directly after, or even the next day, can make a world of difference.

I had another student who was a tennis addict. She was in her mid-forties and had played serious, aggressive tennis three to four times a week for years. The effect of all those games was causing her so much pain in the upper hamstrings and gluteal muscles that she had to drive around town with ice-cold soda cans under her thighs and butt just so she could sit in the car on the way home from the club. My initial advice was to play less tennis, or a softer game. Her response was "No way!" Her social life was heavily tied into her tennis game, and she felt that the personal satisfaction of playing hard and well overrode the pain she experienced afterward. The yoga solution to her pain and her fear of not being able to play her kind of tennis was simpler than either of us thought possible. Every day she did about 15 minutes of warm-up yoga before playing and then another 10 minutes of much lighter and softer cool-down yoga in the changing room immediately after playing. In no time she could enjoy her life after playing tennis—and was spending a lot less money at the soda machine!

I encourage all of you to keep up with your morning yoga practice, to whatever extent is useful, as a preparation for and recovery from the other physical activities you already do and enjoy. Yoga is not exclusive and is helpful in supporting any activity we do. To support physical activities such as tennis, golf, surfing, hiking, swimming, or any other physical or recreational activity that gives you pleasure, try choosing one of the 15-minute yoga practices as a warm-up to ensure that you don't injure yourself and then a lighter 15-minute practice as a cool-down to avoid stiffness and muscular tension resulting from the exertion of the activity. See how it feels and enjoy yourself fully.

How to Use the Practices in the Book

To successfully use the techniques and practices presented in this book to individualize your yoga, observe and respect the breath and body, flowing at your own pace rather than struggling against perceived limitations. Going forward in this spirit, we will progress freely and embody our yoga. Keep in mind that some asanas or vinyasas may be appropriate for you, whereas others are not. This flexibility in perceiving and accepting what actually constitutes yoga for ourselves and others is known as *viniyoga*, or the appropriate individualized application of the tools of yoga.

To individualize your yoga, ask yourself the following questions so that you can understand how to make safe, sensible, and rewarding choices in your morning yoga practice.

1. What is your level of experience with yoga?
2. What is your current level of fitness?
3. What is your level of health?
4. How much time do you have to practice every morning? Every week?

Make note of your answers, and later in the book it will be easier to choose an appropriate starting point and continually progress as your level of experience develops and your needs change. The book will provide clear instructions to help you get started, choose an initial yoga sequence, and progress through continued practice. Once you begin yoga practice, the more consistent you are, the better. The benefits of yoga—increased strength, flexibility, focus, relief of chronic and acute ailments, and a sense of peace—are cumulative. You can experience them only through consistent practice. Try to practice every morning if possible, but no less than three times a week.

2

Morning Energy and Readiness

In the last chapter we discussed breathing techniques, basic spinal anatomy, yoga philosophy, asanas, and pranayamas. With this understanding, we've laid a wonderful foundation for yoga practice. Let's now translate these ideas into your morning practice. Every day we awake and get out of bed, sometimes fresh, alert, and ready to start the day, other times not, depending on our mood and life circumstances. By reading this book you have chosen to start your morning with a fresh perspective and a commitment to working out. In no time at all your morning yoga practice will feel like second nature. One of my yoga teachers used to say, "Yoga should be as regular as brushing your teeth or taking a shower." Can you imagine not brushing your teeth or taking a shower? Of course not! Morning yoga is the time to clean up our energy by engaging ourselves physically at the start of the day. This chapter will provide suggestions concerning when to wash up, go to the bathroom, and engage in activities like reading, phone calls, and e-mail, as well as what and what not to eat and drink and how much. We will also discuss integrating your morning workout into the lifestyle and living space you share with family and pets. Finally, we'll look at equipment, props, atmosphere, and music you can use for your practice and at how to start out and finish up.

Sleeping and Waking Up

The amount and quality of our sleep is as important as the quality of our waking time. The amount of sleep we need varies from person to person. Whereas some people need eight hours of solid sleep every night, others can function healthily on five or six hours. You must determine how much sleep you really need to wake feeling healthy and rested and arrange your evening and nightly routine around ensuring you can get it. Avoid invigorating activities that stimulate the body and mind, staying on the computer into the night, and watching violent or disturbing movies or television before going to sleep. Wind down an hour or two before you actually go to bed by lighting some candles, reading, and having a cup of herbal tea or warm milk. Perform some light breathing exercises like the ones in the last chapter or do some seated meditation in a quiet space. These rituals create a buffer between the events of the day and your sleep time, allowing your body, mind, and spirit to release so that a fully relaxed and deep state of sleep can occur naturally.

Wake up early enough to get in some practice. Try to do at least 20 minutes of yoga; practice longer when you have the time. It's better to be well rested and choose a yoga practice that allows for an unrushed experience that feels fully satisfying, even if you have only 20 minutes. Consistency, quality of practice, and intention are more important than the quantity of practice, because the benefits of yoga accumulate.

Once the alarm goes off, or you wake naturally, take a moment to acknowledge the new day and the rising of the sun. Bringing consciousness to our rising by acknowledging our relationship to the energy of the sun helps us approach each day with fresh anticipation and renewed vigor. It's easy to fall into patterns of negativity reinforced by routine and the burden of our responsibilities. Notice whether your thoughts immediately go to what you have to do throughout the day or to whatever worries or challenges you anticipate. Acknowledge that tendency and bring your thoughts back to the immediate experience of exactly where you are and how you feel on waking. Listen to the sounds around you and open your eyes, bringing mindfulness to your rising by taking a moment to embrace the new day before getting out of bed, and note whether you feel a positive change.

Morning Yogic Hygiene

Once you get out of bed, go to the bathroom to relieve yourself and wash up. *Ayurveda*, India's ancient system of natural healing and yoga's sister science, teaches that during sleep our body naturally releases toxins and waste that accumulate on the tongue. My teacher in India insisted that the first thing I was to do after urinating was to gently scrape my tongue and brush my teeth, before drinking water or tea. For this reason I suggest using a tongue scraper. You should be able to purchase a copper or stainless steel tongue scraper at your local health food store or online. Lightly scrape the tongue from the back to the front. Repeat two to three times, spit, and rinse. Then brush your teeth normally. Wash the face with temperate water and natural soap to freshen up. Blow your nose to get rid of any obstructions in the nasal passage. I suggest using a neti pot with a lukewarm mixture of salt water to clear the nasal passages on a regular basis, especially if you have a tendency toward sinus problems. You can also find a neti pot at your local health food store or online.

Respect your normal bowel functions and, if needed, relieve yourself fully at this time. Don't worry if it takes some time and you need a cup of tea or coffee before the urge arises. If you need to go during your yoga practice, do so and come back to the mat when you finish. Yoga practice encourages elimination and usually helps to get things moving in this area.

I encourage people to shower or bathe after yoga practice. I believe the less you do before starting your daily yoga practice, the more likely you are to do the workout. If you strongly feel the need to shower or bathe prior to doing yoga, there is no harm as long as the yoga practice still happens. However, showering after yoga practice allows you to get dressed and sit down to a morning meal fully refreshed. I suggest showering or bathing before eating; resist the temptation to eat immediately after yoga practice. Ayurveda suggests that our digestive fire or agni needs to fully concentrate on digesting our food. Bathing immediately after a meal can deter the body's digestive energies and create fluctuations in body temperature.

Food and Drink

Before yoga practice you should drink eight ounces of water to hydrate the system and encourage natural peristaltic activity. Resist drinking too much because you should stay relatively light and empty throughout the yoga practice. An over-abundance of food or liquid in the stomach will create a feeling of sluggishness and possibly nausea and indigestion.

I find it useful and often necessary to drink some water, a cup of tea, or both before doing yoga (coffee drinkers, don't worry—this includes you too). The liquid quenches the thirst and gives an energy boost prior to doing yoga. For many of you it may also be useful to get the bowels moving so that you can fully relieve yourself before getting started. Keep in mind that tea and coffee are stimulants but also have diuretic effects. For this reason I suggest limiting yourself to one cup of either (not both) before doing yoga practice, to stimulate the system with energy and help you bring a sense of alertness to the yoga mat. However, drinking tea or coffee is not required if you feel it is unnecessary. A glass of water or fruit juice is sufficient to hydrate and get started in yoga practice. In fact, drinking fruit juice before the morning yoga workout is a great idea. The juice not only hydrates the system but also helps balance the blood sugar. A bit of milk in tea or coffee is fine, but refrain from drinking a full glass of milk before the yoga workout. It may cause a buildup of mucus, impinging on the breath and on a sense of clarity.

Sweating during the workout is good because it helps open the pores and cleanse the system. Because of this sweating, you may need to replenish your hydration during your workout. Sip water as needed throughout the workout or have a glass of water after finishing to replenish fluids. Resist chugging or gulping water during or directly after the workout. Doing so can result in nausea or indigestion related to doing forward bends, twists, and especially inversions like the headstand and shoulder stand during the morning yoga workout. Being mindful in our actions on the yoga mat as well as in how we eat and drink before, during, and after is all part of the practice itself.

I strongly recommend not eating anything before doing yoga in the morning and waiting at least one to two hours after a meal if you practice yoga later in the day. Food that's freshly in the stomach needs time to digest and move down into the intestinal tract. The movements associated with yoga are more comfortable and effective when you do them on an empty stomach. Practicing yoga asanas right after a meal can actually cause indigestion. Of course, you are free to experiment, but don't say you weren't warned! That said, if low blood sugar is an issue, please respect your needs. Eat a piece of fruit or something very light to stabilize your blood sugar and eliminate or minimize any risk of a sudden dip in blood sugar while practicing yoga. If a drop should occur, rest and take some light food or drink to stabilize the blood sugar before resuming yoga practice.

Once you have finished yoga and bathed, sit down and eat some breakfast. Make nourishing and healthy food choices that allow you to retain the benefits of your yoga practice. What food should we eat as a postworkout morning meal? Many different ideas exist as to what is a correct yogic diet. My personal motto about food, which is most certainly informed by yoga practice, is "Tread lightly but take what you need." Many believe that all yogis must be vegetarians for both health and ethical reasons. Many people, however, whether because of genetics, upbringing, or lifestyle, choose not to (or cannot) be vegetarians. Being a vegetarian is not a prerequisite to doing yoga or being a good yogi. We can choose to eat a full spectrum of foods in a nondogmatic way that brings mindfulness to our diet. The questions to ask are these: What foods are healthy? What foods make us happy, and why? Are we harming ourselves or others by eating, or not eating, certain foods?

The food you eat directly after finishing your morning yoga workout and bathing should be nourishing and grounding, yet light. In time, the yoga practice will inform the types of food you intuitively desire. After doing yoga and bathing, you will feel alert and clean. The foods you choose should give you energy and sustenance, without weighing you down. In warmer climates and seasons I suggest eating a bowl of whole-grain cereal or granola and fruit with organic milk (or with soy or rice milk, if you do not eat dairy). In colder climates or seasons I suggest a bowl of hot cereal or oatmeal sweetened with syrup. For nonvegetarians, an organic egg, hard-boiled or scrambled with olive oil, and whole-grain toast are good sources of protein to start the day with. Vegetarian sausages or soy-based fake bacon (fakon) make a nice complement. On occasion, but not daily, treat yourself to something more decadent like a bagel with cream or soy cheese, smoked salmon and fresh tomato, or a decadent baked good. Other good postworkout choices include fresh fruit with organic yogurt or kefir, which help maintain intestinal health. Avoid overly fattening or oily foods like pork products, meat, and heavy cheeses. These foods will dampen the sense of clarity and lightness gained through yoga practice. Try to eat only natural or organic foods and avoid all processed and chemically refined foods. These include fast food, donuts, sodas, and high-sugar pastries. We are completely aware of the toxicity of these processed foods, which are high in fat and refined sugars, to our long-term health and well-being.

To complement our sensible food choices I suggest using a few food-based supplements to maintain and support health. First, you can easily add flaxseed oil to your morning cereal as a source of omega-3 fatty acids and antioxidants, to keep the body juicy and the immune system strong. Second, I suggest using an Ayurvedic supplement called *chywanprash*, a foodlike tonic that looks and tastes like a sweet thick jam. It is completely safe for general use, rich in iron, and full of Indian herbs to promote vitality, virility, strength, and immunity. It is rich in vitamin C from the main ingredient, *amalaki*, the Indian gooseberry. You can purchase it online through several Ayurvedic distributors, and I suggest taking a tablespoon after your morning meal. I consider this supplement to be my Ayurvedic multivitamin.

When eating, sit down, chew well, and be conscious of each bite. Yoga becomes a practice on and off the mat by bringing awareness to every activity, including how, when, and what we eat. All too often in our fast-track society we stuff ourselves on the run. Allow yourself just five minutes to really enjoy whatever you choose for breakfast. How much and how fast you eat is almost as important as what and when. Please be mindful that the portion size is enough to nourish and sustain you until lunch. Eating too much too quickly can easily reduce the digestive and metabolic benefits we gain through yoga practice. Ayurveda suggests that the portion size of any meal should be about the same as the amount you can hold within two cupped hands. That being said, please use a real bowl for cereal (just kidding). By chewing well and eating slowly, we can ensure that we properly digest and absorb the food we eat. Doing so will also make the meal itself into a yogic exercise in mindfulness and bring more pleasure to each bite. Please eat something, and a reasonable amount. I cannot express how unyogic it is to starve yourself of the necessary nutrients that sustain a healthy, happy life. Self-acceptance is just as important a part of yoga as self-development. Continuous fasting or denying yourself the necessary food after doing strenuous activity like yoga is harmful and dangerously depleting.

Workout Space and Equipment

Create a space for your morning yoga workout that can help support the spirit of your desire to improve your physical fitness, mental and emotional well-being, and spiritual connectivity. This space should exist within your own home so that you can get to your morning yoga practice easily at the start of the day. The space should be an optimal setting for the ritual of the practice of yoga and should be as spacious and free of clutter and distractions as possible. However, you must work within the space that you have available and do so in harmony with your family and pets so that everyone in your household can easily respect and support your desire to practice yoga every morning.

- **Physical space.** To practice yoga all you really need is a yoga mat and a clean, quiet space. For some this space may be an entire room dedicated to yoga and meditation, complete with props, blankets, bolster, straps, block, and cushions. For others it may simply be the space next to the bed or between the couch and coffee table. In general you should have enough room for the length of the yoga mat and enough room to the sides to take the arms and legs out wide without hitting anything. Regardless of its size or location, find a way to make this space special for you. Reduce any clutter in the area to cultivate a sense of calm within yourself. Some people enjoy creating a sacred space with devotional items and pictures of loved ones or teachers. Whatever your beliefs, feel free to create a personal altar that gives you peace and inspires and reflects your inner spirit. In warmer climates or during summer months, try taking your yoga mat outside onto a deck or into a garden and enjoying the morning sun close to nature. No matter where, how big, or how small it is, make your yoga space special, reflecting deep commitment to yourself and your well-being. I have often found that once we begin in morning practice we develop a deeper connection to our surroundings. This connection will inherently inform our choices in how we live, often gravitating toward less clutter. In this way our external environment reflects our inner calm.

- **Air and light.** If possible, choose an area with fresh air and morning light. Plants and flowers are nice too. A space full of natural light allows us to absorb and benefit from the morning sun. Fresh air and plants provide a connection to nature and an environment rich in fresh oxygen. Light, air, and a connection to nature are good for the spirit and conducive to a fully uplifting experience that, in combination with endorphins released during the workouts, can help alleviate symptoms of depression. If you have limited access to light or fresh air in your available space, I suggest getting an air purifier to ensure that the air you breathe is free of harmful environmental toxins. For an artificial source of light you can easily and cheaply purchase ultraviolet lamps or bulbs, which provide a beneficial spectrum of light that can also serve as a light source for growing plants, thus infusing the space with a naturally rich source of oxygen and an essential connection to nature. If the space is overly noisy, you can purchase a nature-sounds machine or a small artificial waterfall, both of which can dampen external noise and give you a deepened sense of a naturally relaxing environment.

- **Music.** Some people enjoy light music, whereas others find it a distraction. Either is fine, depending on your mood. Just be sensitive that the music does not interfere with your connection to the breath and body by drawing your attention outward to external stimuli. Often I refrain from using music so that I can bring my focus inward to the body, breath, mind, and spirit. But at times playing music is light and fun and helps create an atmosphere conducive to a relaxed but engaging morning yoga workout. I suggest using music that uplifts your spirit, depending on your personal taste. Experiment with both using and not using music during your morning yoga workout and allow your state of mind to dictate whether or when (and what kind of) music will best help you create an atmosphere conducive to enjoying your daily ritual of morning yoga. Do refrain from types of music that overwhelm your ability to stay connected to body, mind, and spirit by being overly abrasive or stimulating. Yoga is different from cardio workouts in that the breath, not the music, should drive the pacing of the movements within the workout itself. If your available practice space has external noise that can be disruptive, music can help create an environment more conducive to a satisfying yoga practice.

Once we choose an area that is spacious, clean, and quiet, with natural light and fresh air, we need to have some basic equipment on hand for the practice of yoga exercises. One of the many things I love about yoga is its simplicity. To do yoga it is not necessary to have much in the way of space or equipment. But we do need just a few things to support our practice. The following is a basic yoga prop list:

- **Yoga mat.** This is the most essential item on the list. The yoga mat is where all the magic happens. There are many yoga mats on the market to choose from. I suggest looking at a few and determining which thickness and texture feels right for you. Substituting a general exercise or Pilates mat is not an ideal option because of the need for the appropriate length and stickiness that allow us to grip the mat and hold certain postures without slipping. Mats can range in price anywhere from $20 to $60, depending on the brand, the thickness, and the material from which the mat is made. For some people, buying a yoga mat made of environmentally degradable material is a priority. For others, the important factors may be price, comfort, or color. Mats are easy to care for. Every few weeks, simply wash the mat in a machine with soap and water. You can tumble dry it or hang it to dry, depending on the material from which it is made.

- **Mexican blanket.** A Mexican blanket is the second prop for a morning yoga workout. The blanket is essential for support in kneeling, lying, seated, and inverted postures to protect the spine, joints, and connective tissues from injury as a result of the pressure of the hard surface of the mat and the floor.

- **Cushion.** In addition to the Mexican blanket, I suggest purchasing a cushion or zafu (or even a chair, if necessary) for seated meditation and pranayama. It will allow you a comfortable base of support so that you can sit upright easily and avoid discomfort of the hips, sacrum, and lower back.

- **Wooden or foam block.** One or two wooden or foam blocks are extremely useful for providing a higher base of support in challenging and adapted yoga postures. Wooden blocks are heavy and sturdy, whereas foam blocks are lighter but tend to hug the surface of the floor or mat more easily.

- **Strap.** I suggest purchasing a yoga strap for assisting standing, sitting, and lying yoga asanas and stretches so that you can fully experience the physical and energetic expression of the pose while progressing to a level of experience at which the use of a strap is no longer necessary.

Awareness and Dealing With Distractions

Becoming distracted from yoga practice happens easily. Life has a way of getting in front of itself, and it often feels as if we must wake up and jump directly into the hustle and bustle, without a moment for ourselves. This is when our yoga is both most challenging and most needed. As I've stated earlier, I encourage all of you to focus on quality over quantity and length of practice. Work it into your life and reap the many rewards yoga has to offer. Even if your practice feels mundane one day or you begin to plateau, there is a cumulative lasting benefit to the simple participation in breath and body. In time you will break through to a new experience or realization.

The ancient teaching of the yoga sutras states the need to stay focused, committed, and consistent in yoga practice for a long time so that we can move through the fluctuations of life with grace, in playful exploration. The ancient teachings acknowledge the tendency to start yoga practice with strong enthusiasm and warn against the tendency to give up practice as that initial enthusiasm wanes. It's too easy to get out of bed and turn on the television or radio, with the intention of doing yoga later, or to put it off until tomorrow. It's all too tempting to check e-mail, go online, or read the newspaper, telling yourself you'll do yoga right after, only to find that too much time has passed and you have to rush to get out the door. Resist the temptations—the distractions will all be waiting for you when you are done. Most likely you will not have missed a thing by taking some time for your yoga. The world is there, and it will continue to function through your workout; if you hold off from getting caught up in the media blitz and technology, perhaps it will even get a little better because of the contribution of your renewed positive perspective. Allow yourselves this morning time to cultivate inner peace so that when you do engage in the world for work or family, you are more centered and energetic.

Don't get too hung up if you are interrupted or have to take care of obligations when they occur. It's not yogic to get stressed out or angry at spouses, children, or external factors that are beyond your control. I have known many yoga enthusiasts who insist on their quiet yoga time and space with an iron fist. I'm sure my wife would agree that at times I've been guilty of this myself. Maintain a playful attitude with your yoga; this approach will evoke the interest and support of your family and pets. In time you may be surprised to find that you are practicing your morning yoga in good company. For many years I enjoyed the company of my dog Blossom as she sat quietly on the edge of my yoga mat and at times joined in postures with me. For those of you with children, I think playfulness is doubly important, since most kids will not sit so quietly all the time. You may have to kindly ask your children to respect your space and time, invite them to play alongside quietly, or encourage them to join in. You can get creative at including them in the practice of certain postures. In this way, morning yoga becomes a welcome part of the day for both you and your loved ones.

Now that we have discussed tips for yogic hygiene, eating, drinking, and sleeping; where to do your morning workout; and what you require to practice yoga, let's bring these lessons to the mat and allow the practice of yoga to unfold. In time, your intuition combined with the information you have will compose a daily ritual around your morning yoga workout that feels deeply engaging and satisfying. I promise that it will become one of your most coveted and favorite activities in life. So wake up, go to the bathroom, wash up, have some water, tea, or coffee, and then roll out the yoga mat and get ready to practice.

Before starting, check in with the breath and body to evaluate how you feel. From this place of conscious connectivity with yourself you can determine from day to day which yoga practice best suits your current needs. Notice any tension or tightness and the quality of your energy. Your muscles will be tight because of the inactivity of the night's sleep. The yoga workouts are designed to warm up the body, lengthen the muscular systems, and allow you to move gradually and deeply through each pose and sequence. Follow the lesson plans so that you are sufficiently prepared for more intensive asanas and vinyasas. Then move through the necessary counterposes to finish your yoga workout fully balanced and restored.

Determine how much time you have for that day so that you can complete your yoga practice and morning routine free of unnecessary stress. I think it's better to do a full shorter practice than to perform half, or only part of, a longer one. Your yoga practice should feel complete. I suggest setting an intention for the day's practice. Perhaps you want to flow freely, address a specific physical need, work through emotions, or mentally prepare for the day ahead. While doing your yoga, be mindful of your thoughts and stay present on the mat, in your body and breath. Work through life issues by allowing thoughts to arise and then go away while you do asanas, without letting these thoughts overshadow your awareness and your ability to be present in the physical yoga. Please resist imposing unreasonable expectations on your ability to concentrate as a measure of your progression in yoga. We all have ups and downs, good days and less good days. These fluctuations are often reflected in our yoga practice. Yoga is a tool that allows us to move through these mental and emotional fluctuations with grace and fluidity. Enjoy the highs, magic moments, and insightful realizations that occur during and as a result of your daily morning yoga practice.

At the end of your yoga practice, take a moment to rest and then check in and observe your body and state of mind. Fully experience and appreciate the fruit of the practice gained through your efforts before engaging in the rest of our day. Cherish and fully absorb the vibrant energy and the quiet calm within yourself.

3

Yoga Warm-Ups

The heart of the morning yoga workout is saluting the sun. The sun salutations are a series of linked yoga asanas done sequentially to bring intention to the start of the yoga practice and to warm the body, muscles, connective tissues, and joints so that we are safely prepared to move forward into some of the more challenging yoga exercises that will follow. In India these sun salutations were traditionally done at or before sunrise at the beginning of yoga asana practice, while facing east. Each variation of the sun salutation, *surya namascar*, links a series of movements to the breath with the intention of building heat and energizing the body, mind, and spirit. The sun salutations, not unlike warm-up exercises for almost any physical activity, address the spine and almost every muscular system by going through a full range of movements for several repetitions, to ensure that the body is engaged and prepared to move forward into the next activity. The difference between the sun salutation and other types of warm-up activity is that the sun salutations are in themselves a complete workout. They should be fully engaging and fun to do, rather than something to get through in order to get to the real activity at hand. There are mornings when doing a few series of your chosen sun salutation is all you have time for. Doing just that is a perfect choice for a very short morning yoga workout that will certainly bring a benefit, without risk.

The variations of sun salutations that I will present in this book are known as *mandala vinyasas*. Mandala vinyasas are fully balanced circular sequences that start and finish with the same asana, or posture. Like all yoga practice, the sun salutations should be done in such a way that the practitioner can maintain a conscious link and quality of breath and movement throughout the vinyasa. Sun salutations are the perfect start to a morning yoga workout because they are very brmhana in nature and are intended to energize the system, boost the heart rate and circulation, and increase heat to warm you up for the other asanas and vinyasas to come in the practice. It's good to break a sweat; however, if the quality and link between breath and movement is lost, you must examine whether the particular variation of the sun salutation is appropriate for you at that time. If you find that the breath races and you are not able to synchronize the movements with the breath, take a rest and consider choosing a less strenuous variation until you can practice it with some proficiency. Likewise, if you still feel sluggish during or after the sun salutations, perhaps you should choose a more engaging and challenging variation.

We build a vinyasa step-by-step, from the simple to the more complex and challenging, so that we can truly experience a yoga practice that is appropriate for us. In this way I present several variations of the sun salutations, starting with simple preparatory kneeling vinyasas and moving toward more challenging variations, which include arm strengthening, standing poses, and jumpings. To simplify the vinyasas, the preparatory and simplified kneeling sun salutation variations are initially presented independent of the standing poses. Try them in the sequential order as they appear in the book, not necessarily on the same day, but as you progress in yoga. Once you are comfortable with one variation, move to the next. As you progress, feel free to use the more simplified and preparatory variations any time you want a calmer or more restorative yoga practice. Progression in yoga is not a linear process. It's the ability to use all of the tools of yoga to your benefit as needed and when appropriate.

Kneeling Sun Salutation

The kneeling sun salutation is a great introduction for the novice morning yogi, but it can be enjoyed by yoga practitioners at any level of experience. I like to use it as a starting point for the sun salutation sequences, since the preparatory asanas allow us to build toward more complex variations of sun salutations that include more challenging arm support and standing asanas. The kneeling prep vinyasas, A to D, are intended to prepare for and gradually move toward the full kneeling vinyasas. When you can practice one with proficiency, move to the complete kneeling surya namascar sequence. Respect your personal needs and avoid strain or struggle by maintaining the link between the breath and the body. Use ujjayi, ocean breathing, through the nose—smooth, long, and steady. The movements of the body should be synchronized with, and enveloped by, the breath length itself.

Let's start with the first preparatory vinyasa and gradually progress step-by-step toward completing a full kneeling sun salutation. Place a blanket at the center of the mat to protect the knees for the following series of exercises.

Kneeling Prep A

Beginning from a relatively neutral position in a simple asana, we build the kneeling vinyasa by linking the movements of the torso, hips, and shoulders to the breath. By establishing this foundation of understanding, we can then move forward into the slightly more complex steps toward the full sun salutation.

Start on the hands and knees with the palms flat and the arms in line with the shoulders.

1. Inhale, lift the chest, and look up slightly.
2. Exhale, round the spine, and bring the hips back to the heels in a child's pose (see page 49 for explanation), while relaxing the head to the floor.
3. Inhale and come back up to the hands and knees, lifting through the chest and looking up slightly.

Repeat this movement six times, concentrating on the link between the breath and the movement.

Kneeling Prep B

In this prep variation, we add downward-facing dog (see page 50 for explanation) to build arm strength and increase leg flexibility.

Again start on the hands and knees with the palms flat and the arms in line with the shoulders.

1. Inhale, lift the chest, and look up slightly.
2. Curl the toes under and exhale. Extend through the arms and lift the hips to downward-facing dog position. Spread the hands wide, connecting all the fingers and the entire perimeter of the palm to the floor, and extend upward through the arms and upper back. Drop the heels toward the floor, with knees unlocked or slightly bent, while lifting the hips.
3. Start the inhalation and lower the knees back to the floor, lifting the chest and looking up slightly.
4. Start the exhalation, round the spine, and lower the hips back to the heels in a child's pose, while relaxing the head to the floor.

Repeat the vinyasa six to eight times.

Kneeling Prep C

This variation includes the addition of upward-facing dog (see page 59 for explanation) to open the heart and mobilize the upper chest and shoulders through an assertive backbend. Extension along the front of the body is accentuated while you maintain a strong grounding through the hands, arms, legs, and feet.

Again start on the hands and knees with the palms flat and the arms in line with the shoulders.

1. Inhale, lift the chest, and look up slightly.
2. Curl the toes under and exhale while extending through the arms and lifting the hips into downward-facing dog.
3. Keeping the toes curled under, and with straight but unlocked arms, inhale and pivot forward, lowering the hips and opening the chest into upward-facing dog. Looking up slightly, engage the legs to protect the lower back and resist sinking into the shoulders.
4. Start the exhalation and extend through the hands to lift back into downward-facing dog, while relaxing the chin toward the chest.
5. Inhale and lower the knees back to the floor, while lifting through the chest and looking up slightly.
6. Exhale, uncurl the toes, round the spine, and bring the hips back to the heels in a child's pose, relaxing the head to the floor.

Repeat this vinyasa six times.

Kneeling Prep D

Here we add a kneeling backbend with simple arm movements to open the shoulders and chest and relieve any tension that may have accumulated through the arm-supported asanas and vinyasas we have just completed.

Start in a child's pose with the hands on the lower back, the palms facing upward, and the shoulders relaxed.

1. Inhale and come up to stand on the knees while lifting the arms up the sides and overhead and lifting the chest toward the chin in jalandhara bandha.
2. Exhale and come back to the child's pose, lowering the arms down the sides to place the hands on the lower back, with the palms facing up again.

Repeat the vinyasa six times.

Full Kneeling Sun Salutation Vinyasa

Now that we have experienced step-by-step each of the preparatory vinyasas, we can link these asanas together into the full kneeling sun salutation. This kneeling version of a sun salutation is perfect for acquainting people with linking the breath and movements in exercises that are challenging and engaging, without including transitions to and from standing asanas. The sequence is primarily spinally oriented along the torso as you transfer the base of support from the knees to the hands and the feet. This sequence is useful for building heat and mobilizing the spine, hips, and shoulders, while allowing the practitioner to concentrate on the body's relationship to breath in a simplified manner. Again place a blanket in the center of the mat to support the knees.

Start on the hands and knees, palms in line with the shoulders.

1. Inhale, lift the chest, and look up slightly.
2. Curl the toes under and exhale, extending through the arms and lifting the hips up into downward-facing dog.
3. Keeping the toes curled under, inhale and pivot forward to upward-facing dog, lowering the hips, lifting through the chest, and looking up slightly.
4. Exhale, extend through the arms, and lift the hips to downward-facing dog again.
5. Inhale and lower the knees to the floor, lifting the chest and looking up slightly.
6. Uncurl the toes and exhale, bringing the hips back to the heels in a child's pose and relaxing the head to the floor.
7. Inhale and lift to stand on the knees while bringing the arms up the front of the body and overhead.
8. Exhale and take the arms back down the front of the body bringing the hips back to the heels to return to a child's pose again.

Repeat this full sequence six times.

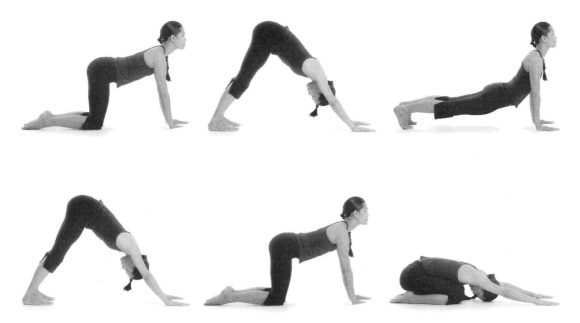

(continued)

(continued)

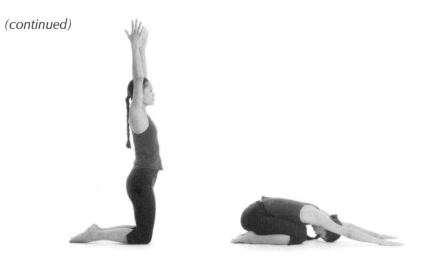

Standing Sun Salutations

Several sequences are commonly recognized as the classic surya namascar, or sun salutation. These sequences add a standing asana to the kneeling sun salutations we have already learned. Here I present three variations of sun salutations you can practice separately, but I also include them within the general yoga practices in coming chapters. As with the kneeling sequences, practice and master the simplified variations before moving on to the more complex and challenging versions. Again, the mind's connection of the breath and body is the primary focus. The ujjayi or ocean breath through the nose should be long, steady, and smooth. The breath should initiate the movements and the movements should reflect the qualities of the breath.

Sun Salutation A

As we already know, many different versions of sun salutations exist throughout the popular styles of yoga. Sun salutation A starts and finishes standing in tadasana, or mountain pose, with the addition of kneeling lunges as a smooth transition between the asanas we have already learned within the kneeling sun salutation.

Stand on the mat gazing forward, arms at the sides, with the feet parallel about hip-width apart.

1. Inhale, gazing up slightly, and lift the arms up the sides and overhead, with the palms facing each other, separate and parallel.

2. Exhale, bending over the legs, and lower the hands to the floor beside the feet, relaxing the neck completely. Bend the knees slightly if needed to allow a natural rounding of the spine, with the weight evenly distributed through the front.

3. On the pause after the exhalation, step the right foot back and drop the right knee to the floor.

4. Inhale, lowering the hips, lift up onto the fingertips, open the chest and look up slightly.

5. Exhale and step the left leg back, dropping the left knee to the floor beside the right and bending the elbows to lower the chest and chin down to the floor.

6. Inhale, lowering the hips and sliding forward, and lift the head, neck, and chest into a low cobra pose (see page 60 for explanation).

7. Curl the toes under and exhale, extending through the arms, and lift the hips into downward-facing dog for one full breath.

8. On the following exhalation, step the right foot forward between the hands.

9. Inhale, lower the hips, lift up onto the fingertips, open the chest and look up slightly.

10. Exhale and step the left foot forward between the hands, with the knees slightly bent and the neck relaxed.

11. Inhale and look up slightly, lifting the arms up the sides and overhead with the palms facing each other, separate and parallel.

12. Exhale and bring the palms together to the heart.

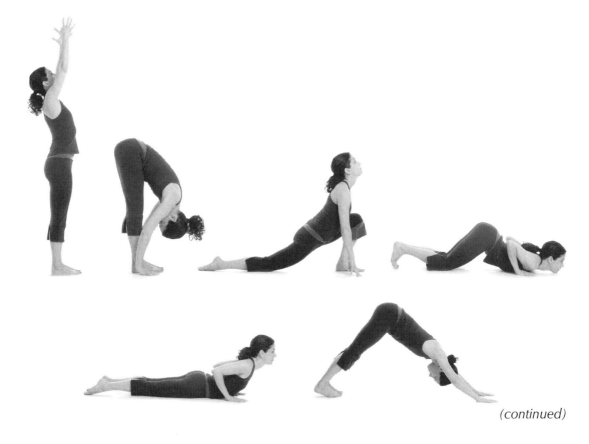

(continued)

(continued)

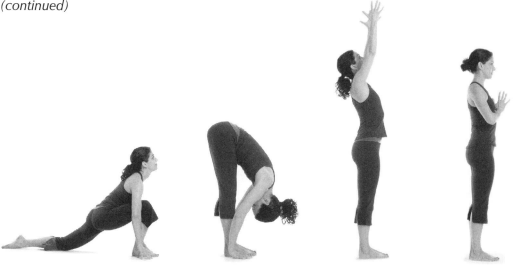

Sun Salutation B

Sun salutation B differs from the previous vinyasas in that we are substituting the kneeling lunges for the warrior pose and the kneeling transition to cobra for the more assertive and challenging *chataranga dandasana*, or stick pose. As we progress in practice we can wake up, warm up, and build up energy, strength, and stamina through these more vigorous, challenging, and complex vinyasas.

Start at the front of the mat with the feet parallel and at hip-width distance and the arms down along the sides of the body.

1. Inhale, lifting the arms up the sides, and bring the palms to meet overhead while gazing up.
2. Exhale, bending over the legs, and place the hands on the floor at either side of the feet, relaxing the neck completely.
3. On the pause after the exhalation, step the right foot back to a long split, placing the right foot forward at a 45-degree angle, and bend the left knee.
4. With a bent left knee, inhale and lift the arms up the sides and overhead into warrior pose (see page 95 for explanation).
5. Exhale, bringing the hands to either side of the left foot, and step back to a plank pose. (Keep the toes curled under with the arms straight and the body extending from the torso through the heels.) Bend the elbows to lower into chataranga dandasana or stick pose (see page 151 for explanation).
6. Inhale and pivot forward into upward-facing dog, gazing up slightly.

7. Exhale and extend through the arms, lifting the hips into downward-facing dog for 4 breaths.

8. Holding the breath out, step the right foot forward between the hands, bend the right knee, and place the left heel down at a 45-degree angle, facing forward.

9. Inhale and lift the arms up the sides and overhead into warrior.

10. Exhale and place the hands to either side of the right foot.

11. Hold the breath out and step the left foot up to meet the right between the hands, bending the knees slightly and relaxing the neck.

12. Inhale, lifting the arms up the sides for the palms to meet above the head, and look up slightly.

13. Exhale and bring the palms together down to the heart.

Repeat the sequence six times, alternating feet each time. On the sixth repetition, stay in warrior pose on each side and in downward-facing dog for 6 breaths.

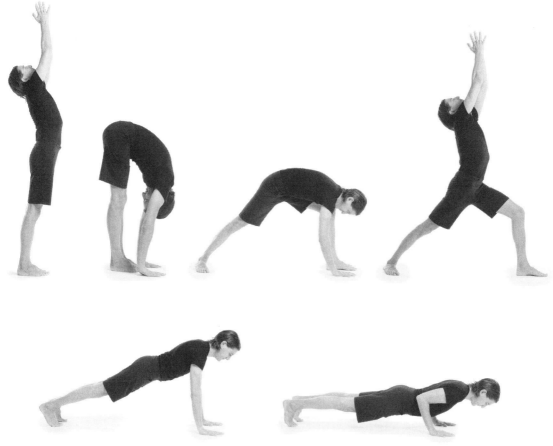

(continued)

(continued)

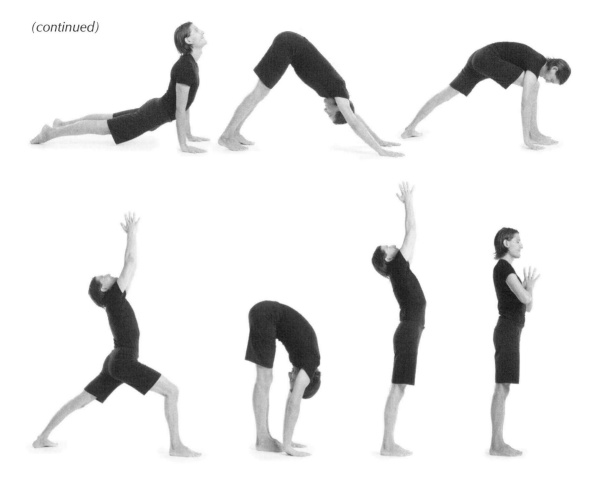

Sun Salutation With Lunge

In this variation of the sun salutation we simply replace the warrior with the standing lunge, or anjaneyasana, which strongly engages the quadriceps muscles of the front leg while stretching the hip flexors of the back leg in an active balancing posture.

Start standing at the front of the mat with the feet together.

1. Inhale and lift the arms up the sides, bringing the palms together above the head and looking up slightly.
2. Exhale and bend over the legs, bringing the palms to the floor at either side of the feet.
3. Hold the breath out and step the right foot back into a long lunge, keeping the back heel and knee lifted off the floor.

4. Inhale and take the arms up the sides to above the head, with the palms separate and parallel, gazing up slightly.

5. Exhale and bend over the right leg, placing the hands at either side of the right foot. Step back into a plank position lower down to chataranga dandasana, or stick pose.

6. Inhale and pivot the hips forward to upward-facing dog, opening the chest and gazing up slightly.

7. Exhale and extend through the arms, lifting the hips back to downward-facing dog and holding for 4 breaths.

8. Hold the breath out and step the right foot forward between the hands into a long lunge, keeping the left knee and heel lifted.

9. Inhale and take the arms up the sides and above the head, gazing up slightly and keeping the palms separate and parallel.

10. Exhale and bend over the front leg, placing the hands at either side of the right foot.

11. On the pause after the exhalation, step the left foot forward to meet the right foot between the hands.

12. Inhale and lift back to standing, looking up slightly and taking the arms up the sides for the palms to meet overhead.

13. Exhale and take the hands together to the heart, relaxing the chin toward the chest.

Repeat this variation of the sun salutation six times, switching legs each time. On the sixth repetition, hold the lunge with the arms above the head for 6 breaths on each side.

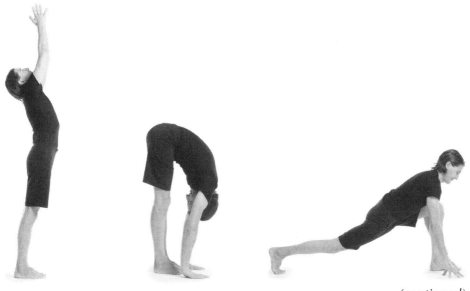

(continued)

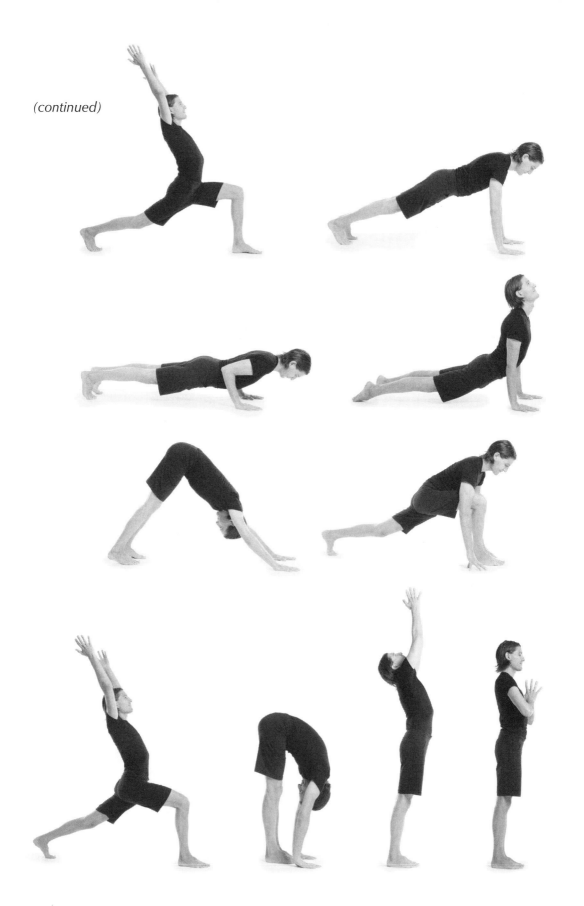

(continued)

Jumping Sun Salutation

This variation of sun salutation includes jumpings. These little leaps of faith are fun, bold, and exhilarating. To do them safely and mindfully, using the breath is central and quite specific in that you do the jumping during the pause after the exhalation. In this way, stability is ensured through mula bandha, or root support in the lower abdominals, which is established during exhalation and maintained after the exhalation, when the jumps are to occur. These jumpings should be done as lightly as possible and with minimal impact. Start at the front of the mat, with the feet parallel and the arms along the sides of the body.

1. Inhale and lift the arms up the sides, bringing the palms to meet overhead and gazing up slightly.
2. Exhale and bend over the legs, lowering the hands to the floor at either side of the feet and relaxing the neck completely.
3. Stay over the legs and inhale, lengthening the spine. Lift the chest to the chin and straighten the arms, coming up onto the fingertips.
4. Exhale and deepen the forward bend, bending the knees slightly and bringing the palms flat to the floor.
5. Hold the breath out and gently hop the feet together back to plank position; inhale.
6. Exhale, bend the elbows, and lower to chataranga dandasana or stick.
7. Inhale and pivot forward to upward-facing dog.
8. Exhale and extend through the arms while lifting the hips to downward-facing dog for 4 breaths.
9. On the pause after the fourth exhalation, gently hop the feet together up between the hands.
10. Inhale and lengthen the spine, lifting the chest to the chin and straightening the arms while coming up onto the fingertips.
11. Exhale and deepen into the forward bend, relaxing the neck.
12. Inhale and lift back to stand, taking the arms up the sides to meet overhead and looking up slightly.
13. Exhale and take the hands together to the heart, relaxing the chin toward the chest.

Repeat the vinyasa five times.

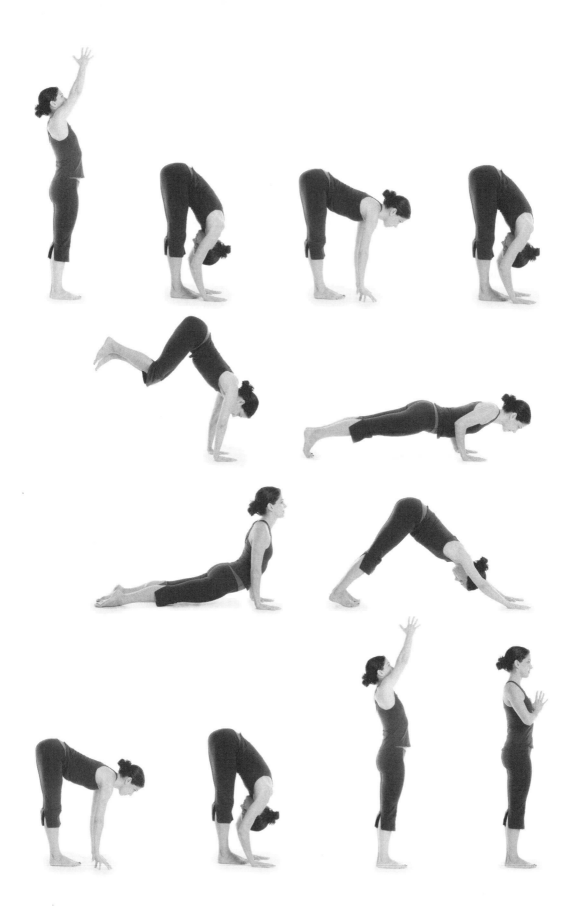

4

Light Practice

Morning yoga workouts can be done by anyone at any age, level of experience, or state of health. Those just getting started in yoga, people with specific health conditions that require a more restorative approach, anyone who lacks sleep or is tired on waking, and people who need to take it easy on a given day but still do some yoga breathing and movement can do these light practices to feel engaged and invigorated. These practices are in no way less substantial or less yogic than the moderate or invigorating workouts. The conscious connection of the breath and the body is truly the heart of the matter; it is represented fully here in a way that will still help you wake up, energize, strengthen, and stretch. I have made subtle adaptations and adjustments to classic asanas to ensure a safe and effective yoga practice. Be aware of sensation and enjoy the work without struggle so that you can fully reap the benefits of the yoga.

Light 15- to 20-Minute Workout

A little of the right yoga done in the right way at the start of the day is a good way to start moving. Either as a first step in the ritual of morning yoga or as a short, light practice on a low-energy day, this workout is the perfect option.

1. Breathing Preparations

Start by lying on the back with the knees bent and the arms along the sides. Relax the body and lengthen the breathing through the nose using ujjayi, or ocean breathing, for 6 breaths.

2. Lying Arm Movements

With the knees bent and both feet flat on the floor, inhale while lifting the arms back overhead. Exhale and take the arms back down along the sides again. Repeat the breath and movements six times. Start each breath a moment before initiating the movement, finishing the movement slightly before the end of the breath.

3. One Knee to the Chest

With the knees bent and both feet flat on the floor, inhale while taking the arms back overhead. Exhale and hug one knee into the chest. Then inhale and return the foot back to the floor as you take the arms back overhead. Repeat the breathing and movements eight times, alternating legs.

4. Lying on Back Legs to Sky (Urdva Prasarita Padasana)

Roll over on the back and hug in the knees, with one hand on each knee. Inhale and take the arms overhead, behind the body, wide enough that the shoulders can connect comfortably to the floor, and extend the legs up, flexing the feet. Exhale, hug in the knees again, and repeat the breath and movements four times. Then hold the position for 6 breaths with the legs extended and the arms back. On the last exhalation, hug in the knees and relax.

5. Lying Twist (Jathara Parivrtti)

Hug both knees into the chest *(a)*. Inhale, extending the arms out to the sides. Then exhale, twisting to the left and lowering both knees to the floor. Inhale, lifting the legs back to center, and then exhale, twisting to the right *(b)*. Repeat the breathing and movement two times to each side. Then stay in the twist to the right and inhale with the arms open wide.

Exhale and take the left hand over and slightly beyond the right hand, extending through the shoulder *(c)*. Inhale and open the left arm again. Repeat the breaths and arm movements four times and then stay in the twist with the arms open for 6 breaths. Inhale, lifting the legs to center, and exhale, twisting to the left. Repeat the breaths and arm movements four times and then stay for 6 breaths on this side. Inhale, lift the legs to center, and hug in the knees.

a

b

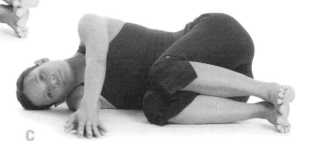

c

6. Bridge (Setu Bandhasana)

Bend the knees with the feet parallel and hip-width apart, comfortably close to the body, and the arms alongside the body *(a)*. Inhale, take the arms back overhead, and lift the hips, grounding through the soles of the feet and lifting the chest toward the chin *(b)*. Exhale, lower the hips to the floor, and take the arms back down from overhead. Repeat the breath and movements four times. Then stay lifted in the bridge for 6 more breaths; inhale, expanding through the chest, and exhale, letting the belly drop in toward the spine. On the final exhale, lower the hips and take the arms back down alongside the body, and relax.

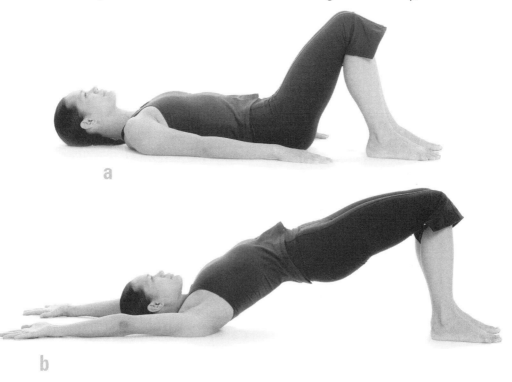

a

b

7. Kneeling Sun Salutation

Kneel on the hands and knees, with the hands in line with the shoulders. Perform the kneeling sun salutation as described on pages 34–36 in chapter 3.

8. Child's Pose (Balasana) to Hero (Virasana)

Start on the knees in child's pose with the forehead relaxed to the floor *(a)*. Inhale and come up to the hands and knees to the hero pose, lifting through the chest and looking up slightly *(b)*. Exhale and come back to child's pose, relaxing the forehead to the floor; repeat the breath and movement six more times.

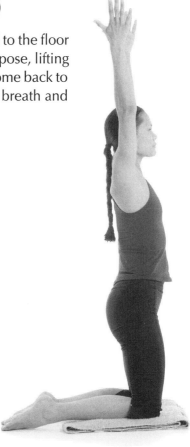

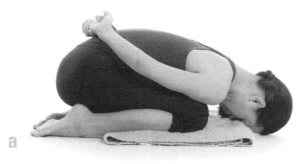

a

b

9. Kneeling Lunge

Kneel on the knees on a blanket for support. Step the left foot forward, place both hands on the left knee, and shift the hips forward. Keeping the hands on the thigh just above the left knee, straighten the arms, lift the chest, relax the shoulders down the back, and stay for 6 breaths. Then shift the weight back, switch legs, and repeat the asana with the right leg forward.

10. Downward-Facing Dog (Adho Mukha Svanasana) and Transition to Stand

Come to the hands and knees. Curl the toes under, exhale through the hands, and lift the hips to downward-facing dog (a). Hold the pose for 5 breaths and then begin to walk the feet forward to the hands, with a relaxed neck (b). Keeping the knees bent slightly and the head, neck, and upper back relaxed, push into the legs and roll up through the spine to stand (c), lifting the head last.

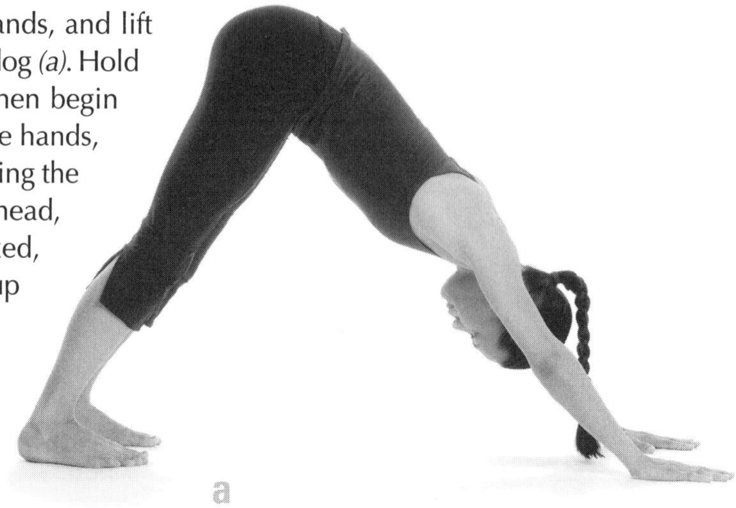

a

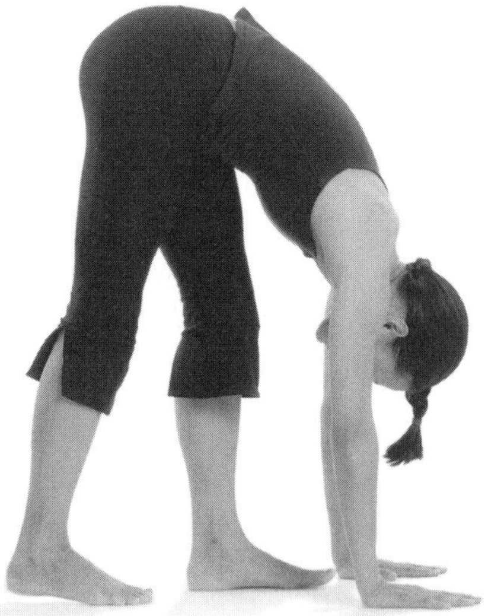

b

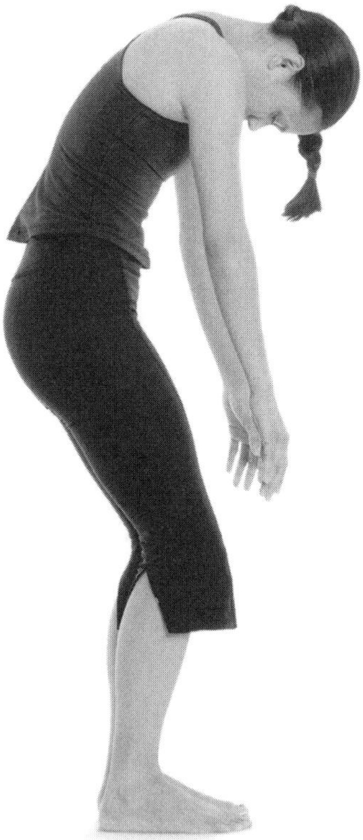

c

11. Mountain (Tadasana)

Stand with the feet hip-width distance apart and parallel and gaze forward *(a)*. Inhale and lift the arms up the sides and overhead with the palms separate and parallel, gazing up slightly *(b)*. Exhale, lower the arms down the sides, and lower the chin down toward the chest. Repeat the breath and movement five more times.

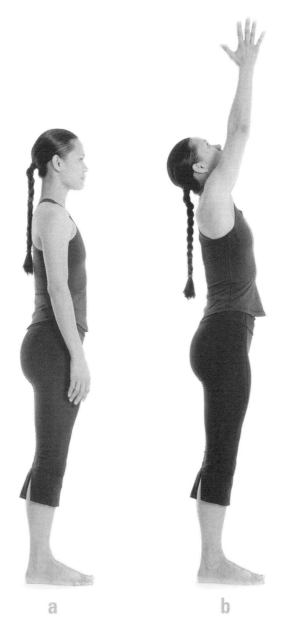

a   b

12. Triangle Twist (Parivrtti Trikonasana) to Standing Split Forward Bend (Prasarita Uttanasana)

Stand in a wide split with the feet parallel and the arms at the sides. Inhale and extend the arms out to the sides (a). Exhale, twist to the right, place the left hand at the floor between the feet, and place the right palm to the sacrum at the very center of the lower back, while gazing up (b). Inhale and lift the back, extending through both arms, then exhale and twist to the left, placing the right hand between the feet and the left palm to the sacrum (c). Inhale while you lift back up to center, extending through both arms.

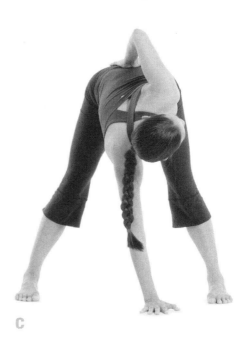

a

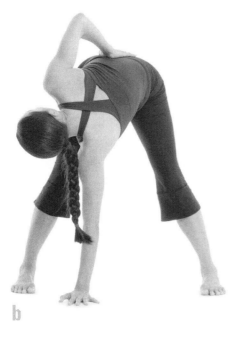

b

c

Then exhale and bend directly forward over the legs, placing both hands on the floor between the feet *(d)*. Inhale and lift back up, extending through the arms. Exhale while you bring the palms together at the heart. Repeat this sequence four times. On the fourth repetition, stay in the twist to each side and in the forward bend split for 6 breaths. Then inhale, lift back to center while extending through the arms, and exhale, bringing the hands together at the heart.

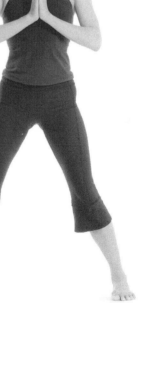

d

13. Finishing Up

With the palms together at the heart, step from the split and bring the feet to the front of the mat. Keeping the palms at the heart, take a moment to notice the breath come and go freely as the chest rises and falls, to integrate your efforts and the benefits of your yoga.

Light 15- to 20-Minute Workout Guide

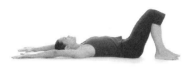

**Breathing Preparations
Lying Arm Movements**

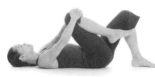

One Knee to the Chest

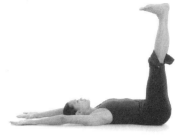

Lying on Back Legs to Sky

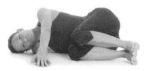

Lying Twist

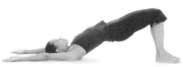

Bridge

**Kneeling Sun Salutation
See pages 35–36**

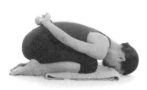

Child's Pose to Hero

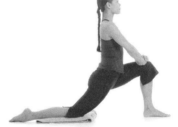

Kneeling Lunge

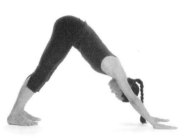

**Downward-Facing Dog
and Transition to Stand**

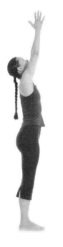

Mountain

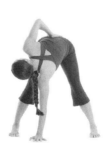

**Triangle Twist to Standing
Split Forward Bend**

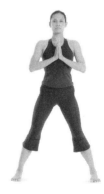

Finishing Up

Light 30- to 40-Minute Workout

The 30-minute light morning yoga workout is designed for novices still adjusting to regular yoga practice and for more experienced practitioners wanting a light workout that feels complete, but not rigorous, at the start of the day. With the increased workout time we have the opportunity to practice a greater variety of asanas and include seated alternate breathing exercises at the end of the practice, for a fuller experience.

1. Breathing Preparations

Stand at the front of the mat with the feet about hip-width apart and parallel, the arms at the sides, and the gaze forward. Bring your awareness to the breath and begin to lengthen the inhalation and deepen the exhalation using ujjayi, or ocean breathing through the nose, for 6 breaths.

2. Mountain (Tadasana)

Stand at the front of the mat with the feet hip-width distance apart and parallel and the arms along the sides (a). Inhale and lift the arms up the sides and overhead (b). Gaze up slightly and leave the palms separate and facing each other, with the shoulders relaxed down the back. Exhale while you lower the arms back down the sides and relax the chin to the chest. Repeat the breathing and movements six times.

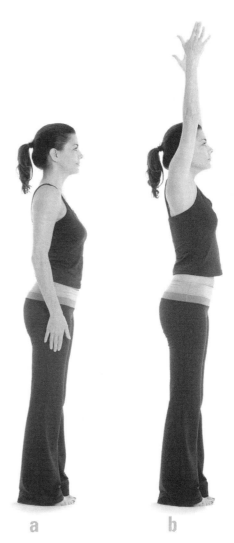

a   b

3. Standing Forward Bend (Uttanasana)

Inhale while lifting the arms above the head, and then exhale, bending over the legs and lowering the hands to the floor. Relax the neck completely and bend the knees as much as needed. Inhale and lift up, taking the arms up the sides and overhead and gazing up slightly. Repeat the breaths and the movements up and down four times. Then stay in the forward bend for 6 breaths; inhale, expanding through the back of the body, and exhale, deepening the forward bend. Inhale again, lifting back up and taking the arms above the head, and exhale as you lower the arms down along the sides and bring the chin toward the chest.

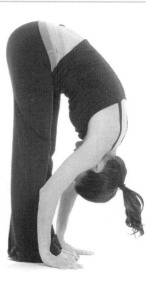

4. Warrior (Virabhadrasana)

With the arms at the sides, stand in a split with the legs four-and-a-half to five feet apart, right leg forward and left leg back. The right foot, hips, and shoulders face forward, and the left foot is turned outward at a 45-degree angle. Inhale, bend the right knee, and lift the arms up the sides and overhead, palms separate and parallel and shoulders relaxed, while also lifting through the chest and gazing up *(a)*. Exhale and lower the arms back down the sides, lowering the chin toward the chest *(b)*. Repeat the breath and movement four times and then stay in warrior for 6 breaths. Exhale and lower the arms back down the sides, straightening the right leg and relaxing the chin to the chest. Switch legs and repeat the posture on the other side.

a

b

5. Triangle (Trikonasana)

Keep the same foot position as in the warrior vinyasa. Open the shoulders to the side. Inhale and lift the arms out, reaching through the hands. Extend forward and exhale, placing the left hand on the left shin and reaching the right hand upward *(a)*. The left or bottom hand should be on the shin high enough for the front of the body to stay open. Straighten the legs, with an unlocked left knee. Inhale feeling the energy ground through the feet and look up, reaching up through the right hand with the palm open and the fingers spread wide. Exhale while lowering the right arm behind the back, turning the head to look down at the left foot and keeping the left arm straight *(b)*. Inhale and extend the right arm up again. Repeat the arm movements four times and then hold the triangle, with the arm extended, for 6 more breaths. Then inhale and lift back up to standing, reaching through the arms. Exhale and lower the arms to relax. Pivot the feet in the other direction and repeat triangle on the other side.

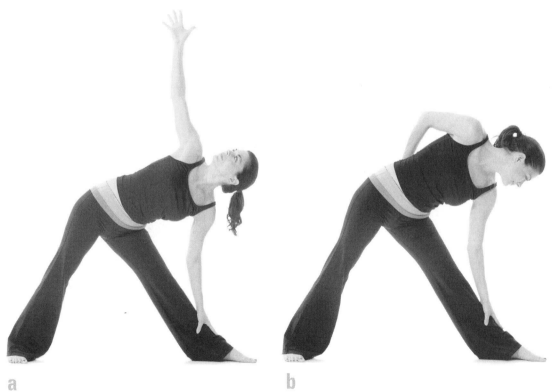

a   b

6. Triangle Twist (Parivrtti Trikonasana)

Stand in the split with the feet parallel. Inhale, extending the arms out to the sides *(a)*, and exhale, twisting to the right, placing the left hand between the feet and the right hand on the sacrum, and looking up *(b)*. You can place the bottom hand directly in the center, toward the inside of the right foot, or on the outside of the right foot for increasing intensity. Remain grounded through both feet while allowing the hips to rotate in the direction of the twist. Bend the leg that is in the direction of the twist slightly if needed, while keeping the far leg straight. If the neck and shoulders feel strained, look down.

Inhale, reaching through the arms, and lift back to center. Exhale and twist to the left, placing the right hand on the floor between the feet and the left hand on the sacrum while looking up. Repeat the breaths and movements, twisting four times to each side. On the fourth repetition, stay in the twist for 6 breaths on each side; inhale, easing up and lengthening the spine, and exhale while deepening into the twist. Then inhale, lifting through the arms back to center, and exhale, relaxing the arms down at the sides.

a

b

7. Standing Split Forward Bend (Prasarita Uttanasana)

Remain in the split with the feet parallel and the arms at the sides. Inhale and lift through the arms. Exhale, bend over the legs, and bring both hands to the floor between the feet, relaxing the neck completely and bending the knees slightly if necessary. Keep some weight distributed through the front of the feet. Stay in the split forward bend for 6 breaths; inhale, lengthening the spine, and exhale, deepening the forward bend. Then inhale, lift back up, and extend through both arms to the sides. Exhale and bring the palms together at the heart.

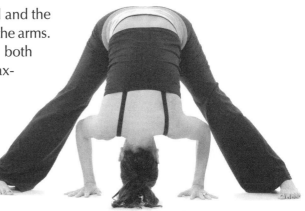

8. Kneeling Upward-Facing Dog (Urdva Mukha Svanasana) to Cobra (Bhujangasana) to Downward-Facing Dog (Adho Mukha Svanasana) to Child's Pose (Balasana)

Place a blanket in the middle of the mat and come to the hands and knees *(a)*. Inhale, pivot forward, and lower the hips to an adapted upward-facing dog, opening the chest and looking up, with slightly bent elbows *(b)*. Exhale, bend the elbows, and lower to the

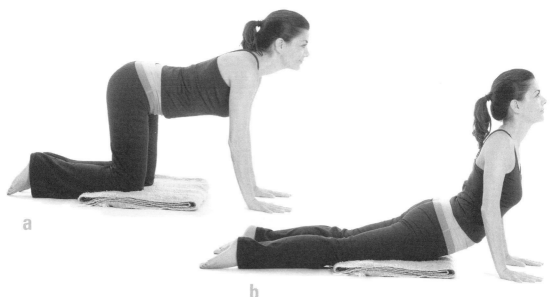

floor (c). Inhale, press into the hands, and lift the head, neck, and chest to cobra (d). Curl the toes under. Exhale, extend through the arms, and lift the hips to downward-facing dog (e), bending the knees as much as needed, lowering the heels to the floor, and relaxing the chin to the chest. Inhale, lower the knees to the blanket, and lift through the chest, looking up slightly. Exhale and come to child's pose (f). Inhale, lift back up to the hands and knees (a), and pivot the hips forward to upward-facing dog (b) to start the vinyasa again. Repeat the vinyasa six times to finish in child's pose.

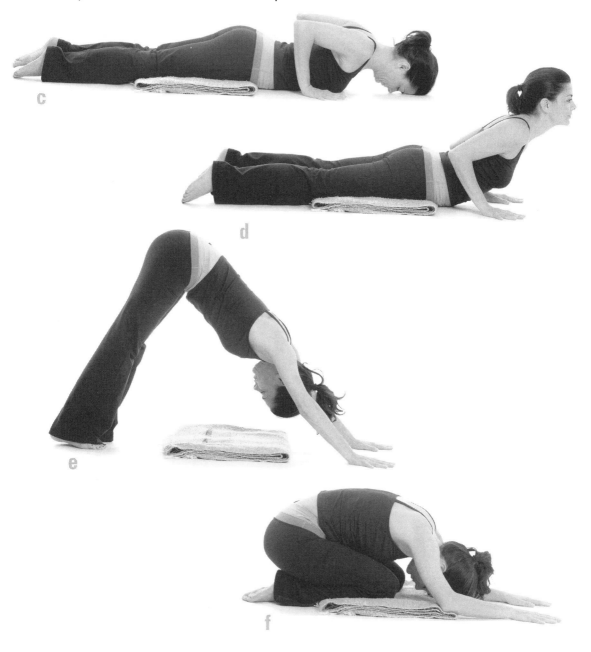

9. Child's Pose (Balasana) to Standing Knees

Start in child's pose with the blanket under the knees and place the hands on the lower back with the palms facing up. Inhale and come up to stand on the knees, taking the arms overhead, lifting the chest, and looking up slightly. Exhale and lower back to child's pose again, bringing the hands to the back. Repeat the breaths and movements six times. Remain standing on the knees and lower the arms down the sides for the next posture.

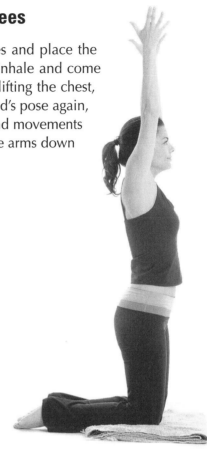

10. Kneeling Lunge

Stand on the knees on a blanket for support, step the right foot forward, and place both hands on the right knee, shifting the hips forward. Straighten the arms, lift the chest, relax the shoulders down the back, and hold for 6 breaths. Then shift the weight back, switch legs, and repeat the asana with the left leg forward.

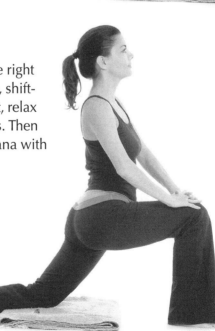

Light 30- to 40-Minute Workout

11. Child's Pose (Balasana)

Bring the hips to the heels, extend the arms in front of the body, and relax the forehead to the floor in a child's pose for 6 breaths.

12. Seated Twist (Ardha Matsyendrasana)

Sit a on a blanket with both legs extended forward. Place the right foot to the outside of the left thigh, leaving the left leg long. Place the left arm along the outside of the right thigh and place the right hand, lifted lightly on the fingertips, on the floor behind the body. Soften the gaze to take the focus inward. Inhale while lifting and lengthening the spine and then exhale, engaging the twist to the right, drawing the belly in and up, and turning the head in the same direction. Be mindful not to strain the spine by forcing through the arms and shoulders. Stay in the twist for 6 breaths and then release; repeat the twist to the left.

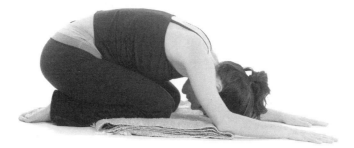

13. Head-to-Knee Forward Bend (Janu Sirsasana)

Sit upright with both legs extended forward. Place the sole of the right foot to the inside of the left thigh, with the right knee out to the side. Pivot the hips forward and inhale, lifting the arms overhead. Exhale and bend over the extended left leg, placing the hands over the top of the right foot. Relax the head toward the left knee, bending the left knee slightly if necessary. Inhale and lift back up, taking the arms overhead. Then exhale and bend over the left leg again. Repeat the breaths and movements four times. Then stay over the left leg for 6 more breaths; inhale, expanding

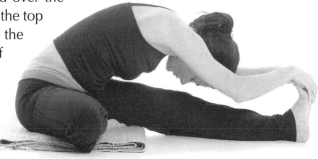

through the back of the ribs, and exhale, deepening the forward bend. Inhale and lift back up, taking the arms overhead, and exhale, lowering the arms. Switch legs and repeat the asana on the other side.

14. Cobbler's Pose (Baddha Konasana)

Sitting upright on the blanket, bring the soles of the feet together in front of the body, close to the groin. Use the hands to open the feet like a book and externally rotate the hips open *(a)*. Holding the feet, inhale and straighten the arms, lengthening the spine. Lower the chin to the chest in jalandhara bandha and stay for 6 breaths, adding a slight pause between the breaths. On the sixth exhalation, round the spine over the legs and extend the arms in front of the body *(b)* for 6 more breaths. Then walk the arms back and inhale, lifting back up again.

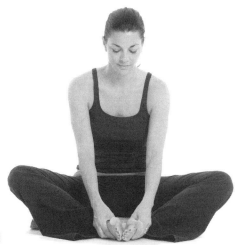

a

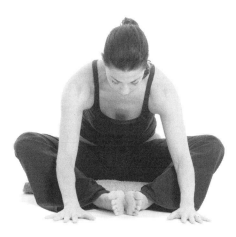

b

15. Bridge (Setu Bandhasana)

Remove the blanket and lie on the back of the body. Bend the knees with the feet parallel and at hip-width, comfortably close to the body, and with the arms alongside the body *(a)*. Inhale, take the arms back overhead, and lift the hips, grounding through the soles of the feet and lifting the chest toward the chin *(b)*. Exhale, lower the hips to the floor, and take the arms back down from overhead. Repeat the breath and movements four times. Then stay lifted in bridge pose for 6 more breaths; inhale, expanding through the chest, and exhale, letting the belly drop in toward the spine.

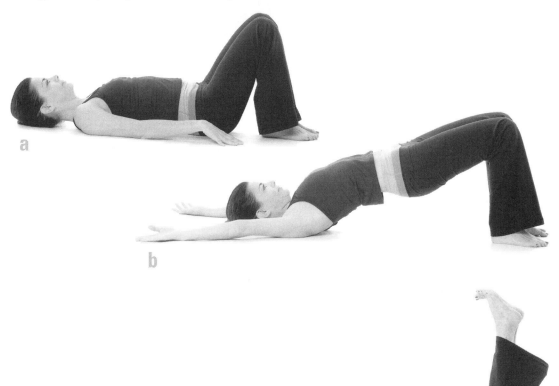

16. Supported Bridge Legs to Sky (Viparitakarani)

Remain lifted in bridge and place a block, horizontally long, under the sacrum. Take the arms back down along the sides. Lift up one leg and then the other so that both legs are extended up with the feet flexed. Stay in viparitakarani for 10 breaths. Then bring both feet back to the floor, remove the block, and lower the hips.

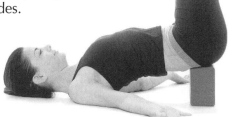

17. Corpse Pose (Savasana)

Straighten both legs. If you wish, you can place a rolled blanket under the knees to support the lower back. Place the arms alongside the body with the palms facing up, close the eyes, release any tension, and relax completely into the corpse pose for several minutes to absorb the effort of the practice.

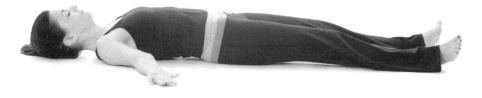

18. Lying Twist (Jathara Parivrtti)

After several minutes in the savasana, hug both knees into the chest. Inhale, extending the arms out to the sides, and exhale, twisting to the left and lowering both knees to the floor. Inhale while lifting the legs back to center and exhale, twisting to the right *(a)*. Repeat the breaths and movements two times to each side. Then stay in the twist to the right and inhale with the arms open wide. Exhale, taking the left hand over and slightly beyond the right hand and extending through the shoulder *(b)*. Inhale and open the left arm again. Repeat the breaths and arm movements four times and then stay in the twist with the arms open for 6 breaths. Inhale, lifting the legs to center, and exhale, twisting to the left. Repeat the breaths and arm movements four times and then stay for 6 breaths on the other side. Inhale, lifting the legs to center, and hug in the knees.

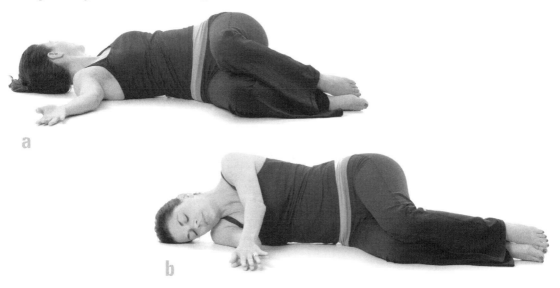

a

b

19. Lying Hip Opener

Lying on the back, with the knees bent and the feet at hip-width distance, place the left ankle on the top of the right thigh and drop the left knee out to the side to open the left hip. Take the right arm around the outside of the right leg and the left arm between the legs, to interlace the fingers on the top of the right shin. Stay for 8 breaths. Then exhale, drawing the legs in toward the body while keeping the head relaxed to the floor, and inhale, easing up slightly. Release the hands and legs and repeat the pose on the other side.

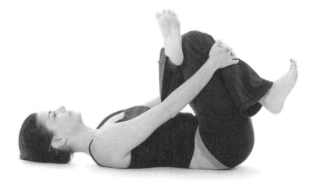

20. Easy Seated Alternate Nostril Breathing (Pranayama)

Come up to an easy cross-legged seated position on the blanket. Extend the right hand forward with the palm facing up. Bring the index and the middle finger into the palm. Then bring the right hand to the nose, placing the ring finger on the left nostril and the thumb on the right, just below the bridge bone. Take one full round of breath (inhale and exhale) through both nostrils. Close off the left nostril completely with the ring finger and inhale through the right. Close both nostrils and hold for a few seconds, then release the ring finger and exhale through left nostril. Inhale through left nostril, close both nostrils, and hold the breath in for a few seconds again. Then release the right nostril and exhale to complete one full round. Repeat this breathing for six full rounds or 12 breaths, finishing with an exhalation through the right nostril. Relax the right hand down, breathe freely, and take a moment to fully experience an energized and peaceful state of being.

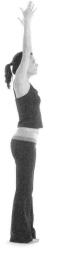

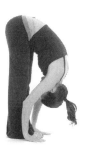

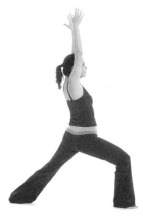

**Breathing Preparations
Mountain**

Standing Forward Bend

Warrior

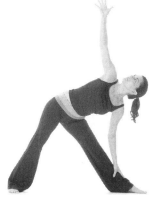

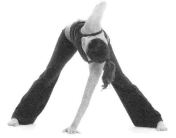

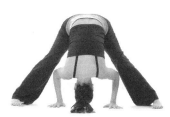

Triangle

Triangle Twist

Standing Split Forward Bend

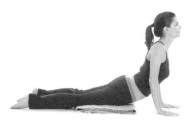

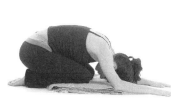

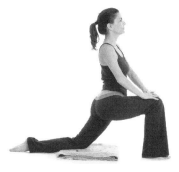

**Kneeling
Upward-Facing Dog Vinyasa
Repeat 6 times**

**Child's Pose
to Standing Knees**

Kneeling Lunge

Light 30- to 40-Minute Workout Guide

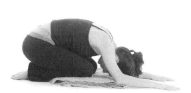

Child's Pose

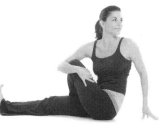

Seated Twist

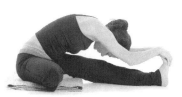

Head-to-Knee Forward Bend

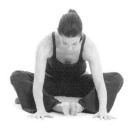

Cobbler's Pose

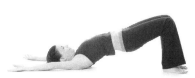

Bridge

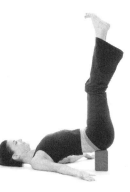

Supported Bridge Legs to Sky

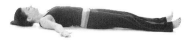

Corpse Pose

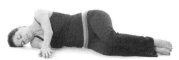

Lying Twist

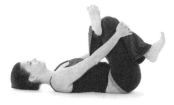

Lying Hip Opener

**Easy Seated Alternate
Nostril Breathing
See page 10**

The 60-minute light practice is an opportunity to have a deep, relaxed, and comprehensively engaging morning yoga workout. Spending more time with a larger variety of asanas and vinyasas will allow you to fully experience the benefits of increased strength, flexibility, stamina, and focus. This practice is just right for any level of experience, as either a longer commitment to regular restorative practice or an indulgent treat on days when your schedule allows.

1. Breathing Preparations

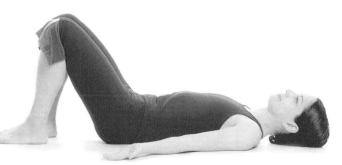

Start by lying on the back with the knees bent and the arms along the sides. Relax the body and lengthen the breathing through the nose using ujjayi, or ocean breathing, for 6 breaths.

2. Lying Arm Movements

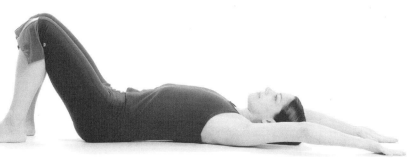

With the knees bent and both feet flat on the floor, inhale and lift the arms back behind the head. Exhale and take the arms back down along the sides again. Repeat the breath and movements six times. Start each breath a moment before initiating the movement, finishing the movement slightly before the end of the breath.

3. One Knee to the Chest

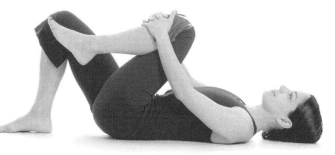

With the knees bent and both feet flat on the floor, inhale and take the arms back overhead. Exhale, hugging one knee into the chest, and inhale, returning the foot back to the floor as you take the arms back overhead. Repeat the breaths and movements eight times, alternating legs.

Light 50- to 60-Minute Workout

4. Seated Arm Stretch

Come up and sit in a cross-legged position with one hand on each knee. Inhale and lift the arms up the sides and over-head. Interlace the fingers and turn the palms to face up *(a)*. Exhale and bend the elbows slightly. Inhale and reach through the palms, straightening the arms and gazing up *(b)*. Exhale, relaxing the posture slightly. Stay in the pose for 6 full breaths. On the last exhale, release the fingers and bring the arms down the sides and back to the knees.

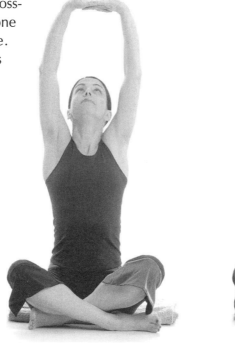

a

b

5. Seated Side Bend

While seated in a cross legged position, take the left hand to the right knee and inhale, lifting the right arm overhead and reaching it toward the left as you bend sideways. Hold the pose for 6 breaths. Then exhale and relax the right arm back down. Repeat the seated stretch on the other side.

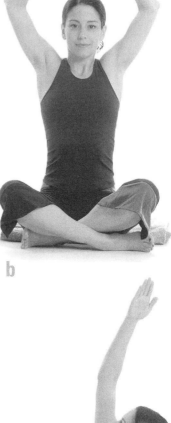

6. Cat to Child's Pose (Balasana) to Downward-Facing Dog (Adho Mukha Svanasana)

Come up onto the hands and knees, placing a blanket under the knees for support. Inhale, lifting the chest in cat *(a)* and looking up slightly, and exhale back to child's pose *(b)*. Inhale and come up to the hands and knees. Curl the toes under you and exhale, extending through the arms and lifting the hips into downward-facing dog *(c)*. Inhale and come back to the hands and knees. Repeat the vinyasa six times. Hold the downward-facing dog pose for 5 breaths on the last repetition, relaxing the chin toward the chest, lifting the hips, dropping the heels, and bending the knees slightly if needed.

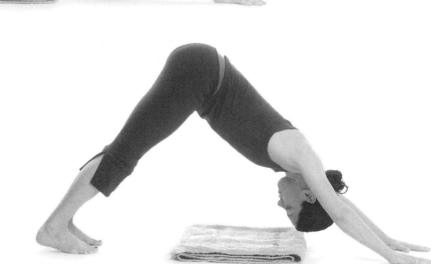

a

b

c

7. Transition to Standing

From downward-facing dog begin to walk the feet up to the hands *(a)* into a standing forward bend, with knees bent slightly and the upper back, neck, and arms relaxed. Push through the feet and roll up through the spine to stand, slowly lifting the head up last *(b)*.

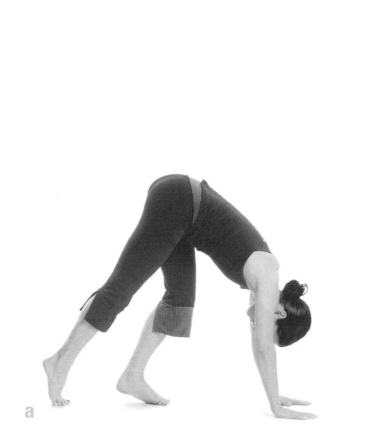

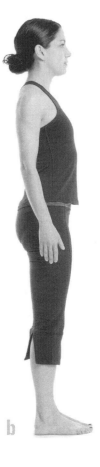

8. Standing Lunge (Anjaneyasana)

Stand at the front of the mat with the feet hip-width apart and parallel, the arms at the sides, and the gaze forward. Inhale, lift the arms up the sides and overhead with palms separate and parallel, and gaze up slightly *(a)*. Exhale, bend over the legs, bringing the palms to the floor at either side of the feet, and step the right foot back, keeping the back heel and knee lifted off the floor *(b)*. Inhale into anjaneyasana pose, lifting the chest and arms overhead and looking up slightly *(c)*. Exhale, place the hands back down at either side of the left foot, and step the right foot forward between the hands. Inhale here and then exhale, stepping the left foot back and keeping the heel and knee lifted. Inhale into the lunge, lifting the chest, taking the arms overhead, and looking up slightly. Exhale, place the hands down at either side of the right foot, and step the left foot forward between the hands. Inhale and lift back to stand, taking the arms up the sides and overhead with the palms separate and parallel and looking up slightly. Exhale and bring the palms together to the heart. Repeat the breathing and movements six times, alternating legs. On the last repetition, hold the lunge for 6 breaths on each side.

9. Warrior (Virabhadrasana)

Stand in a split with the legs four-and-a-half to five feet apart, right leg forward and left leg back, and the arms at the sides *(a)*. The right foot, hips, and shoulders face forward and the left foot is at a 45-degree angle from forward. Inhale, bend the right knee, and lift the arms up the sides and overhead, with the palms separate and parallel and the shoulders relaxed, while lifting through the chest and gazing up *(b)*. Exhale, lower the arms back down the sides, straighten the right leg, and lower the chin toward the chest. Repeat the breath and movement four times and then stay in warrior pose for 6 breaths. Exhale, lowering the arms back down the sides, straightening the right leg, and relaxing the chin to the chest. Switch legs and repeat the posture on the other side.

a

b

10. One-Sided Standing Forward Bend (Parsva Uttanasana)

Staying in the same stance as for the previous warrior pose, inhale and lift the arms up to the sides and above the head, keeping the left leg straight and the gaze forward. Exhale and bend over the straight left leg, placing the hands to the floor (or on blocks) at either side of the left foot. Inhale and lift back up to standing, taking the arms up the sides and overhead, with the palms separate and parallel, and gazing forward. Exhale and bend over the left leg again. Repeat the breathing and movements four times. Stay in the forward bend for 6 more breaths, inhaling while you expand through the back of the body and exhaling while you deepen the pose, ground through both feet, and draw the left hip back with an unlocked left knee. Then inhale and lift back to stand, taking the arms up the sides and overhead, and exhale, relaxing the arms down the sides. Switch legs and repeat the posture on the other side.

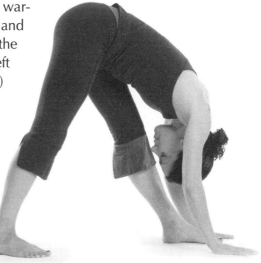

11. Triangle (Trikonasana)

In the same stance as the previous pose, open the shoulders to the side while the hips rotate forward. Inhale and lift both arms out. Exhale and lower the right hand to the right shin, keeping the right leg straight with an unlocked knee. Be mindful that the hand is placed on the shin high enough for the chest and shoulders to remain open. Inhale and extend through the left arm, spreading the fingers wide, while gazing up at the left hand *(a)*. Exhale and take the left arm behind the back, keeping the right arm extended, and look down at the right foot *(b)*. Inhale and lift the left arm back up, looking at the left hand. Repeat the breaths and movements four times and then stay lifted in the triangle for 6 more breaths. If the neck and shoulders feel strained, look down at the right foot while keeping the left arm lifted. Then inhale, extending through both arms, and lift up to stand. Exhale and lower the arms. Switch feet and repeat the trikonasana on the other side.

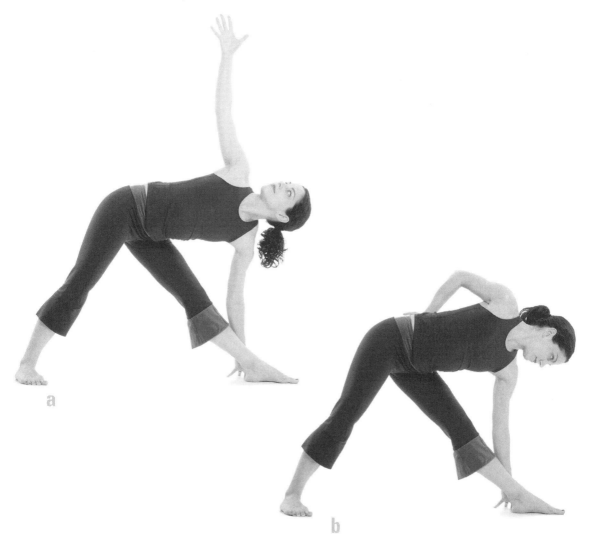

a

b

12. Triangle Twist (Parivrtti Trikonasana)

Stand in the split with the feet parallel. Inhale, extending the arms out to the sides *(a)*. Exhale and twist to the right, placing the left hand between the feet and the right hand on the sacrum, looking up *(b)*. You can place the bottom hand directly in the center, toward the inside of the right foot, or on the outside of the right foot for increasing intensity. Remain grounded through both feet while allowing the hips to rotate in the direction of the twist. Bend the leg that is in the direction of the twist slightly if needed, while keeping the far leg straight. If the neck and shoulders feel strained, look down.

Inhale, reaching through the arms, and lift back to center. Exhale and twist to the left, placing the right hand on the floor between the feet and the left hand on the sacrum while looking up. Repeat the breaths and movements, twisting four times to each side. On the fourth repetition, stay in the twist for 6 breaths on each side. Inhale, easing up and lengthening the spine, and exhale while deepening into the twist. Then inhale, lifting through the arms back to center, and exhale, relaxing the arms down at the sides.

a

b

Light 50- to 60-Minute Workout

13. Standing Split Forward Bend (Prasarita Uttanasana)

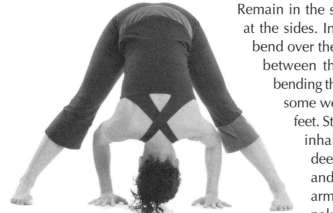

Remain in the split with the feet parallel and the arms at the sides. Inhale and lift through the arms. Exhale, bend over the legs, and bring both hands to the floor between the feet, relaxing the neck completely, bending the knees slightly if necessary, and keeping some weight distributed through the front of the feet. Stay in the split forward bend for 6 breaths; inhale, lengthening the spine, and exhale, deepening the forward bend. Then inhale and lift back up, extending through both arms to the sides, and exhale, bringing the palms together at the heart.

14. Kneeling Upward-Facing Dog (Urdva Mukha Svanasana) to Cobra (Bhujangasana) to Downward-Facing Dog (Adho Mukha Svanasana) to Child's Pose (Balasana)

Place a blanket in the middle of the mat and come to the hands and knees *(a)*. Inhale and pivot forward, lowering the hips to an adapted upward-facing dog, opening the chest, and looking up, with slightly bent elbows *(b)*.

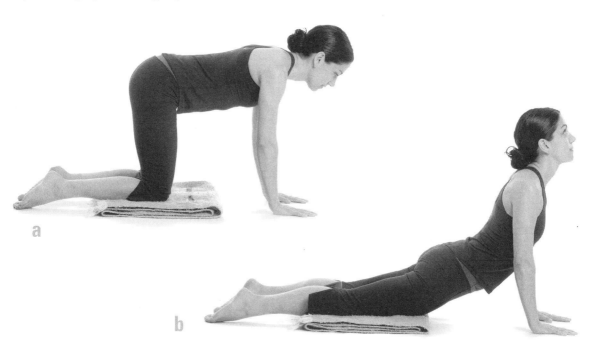

Exhale, bend the elbows, and lower to the floor. Inhale, press into the hands, and lift the head, neck, and chest to cobra position *(c)*. Curl the toes under and exhale, extending through the arms and lifting the hips to downward-facing dog *(d)* (bend the knees as much as needed, lowering the heels to the floor and relaxing the chin to the chest). Inhale and lower the knees to the blanket, lifting through the chest and looking up slightly. Exhale and come back to child's pose *(e)*. Inhale, lift back up to the hands and knees, and pivot the hips forward to upward-facing dog to start the vinyasa again. Repeat the vinyasa six times and finish by bending the elbows from upward-facing dog to lower the body down to the floor.

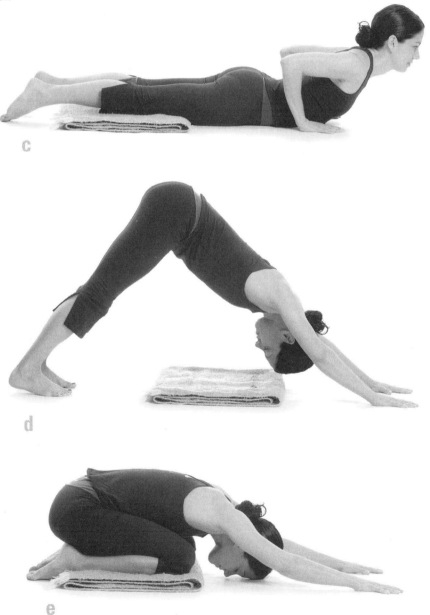

c

d

e

15. Cobra (Bhujangasana)

Lie on the front of the body with the forehead to the floor and the hands placed by the ribs. Inhale, pressing into the hands lightly, and lift the head, neck, and chest up into cobra. Exhale and lower the head, neck, and chest back down. Repeat the breathing and movements four times. Then stay in the cobra pose for 6 breaths; exhale, staying lifted and letting the belly press into the floor, and inhale, lifting through the chest. Then exhale and relax back to the floor.

16. Locust (Salabasana)

Continue lying on the front of the body, taking the arms back along the sides and bringing the palms to face up (a). Inhale, lift the head, chest, legs, and arms, rotating the palms to face down as you lift, and gaze up (b). Exhale and lower the head, chest, legs, and arms back down, rotating the palms to face up. Repeat the breaths and movements four times and then stay in the locust for 6 more breaths.

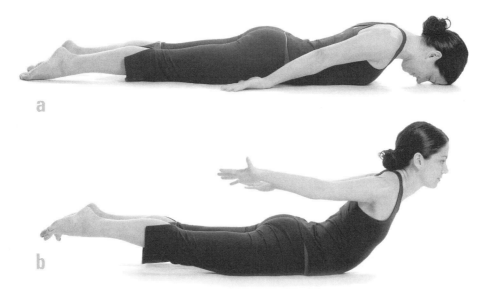

a

b

17. Lying on Back Legs to Sky (Urdva Prasarita Padasana)

Roll over on the back and hug in the knees, with one hand on each knee *(a)*. Inhale and take the arms overhead back behind the body, wide enough that the shoulders can connect comfortably to the floor, and extend the legs up, flexing the feet *(b)*. Exhale, hug in the knees again, and repeat the breath and movements four times. Then hold the position for 6 breaths with the legs extended and the arms back. On the last exhalation, hug in the knees and relax.

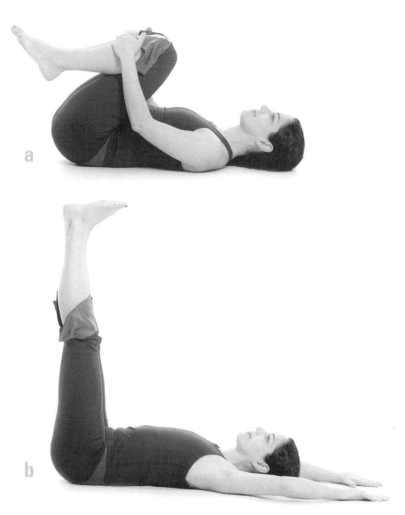

18. Leg Lifts (Urdva Padasana)

Lying on the back, take the arms slightly underneath the body with the palms face down and bend the knees to the chest. Inhale, extend the legs up, and flex the feet. Exhale and hold. Then inhale, lowering the legs about two-thirds of the way to the floor, and exhale, lifting up the legs again and bending the knees slightly at the top of the pose to ease lower-back tension. Repeat the breaths and movements six times and then hold the legs about two-thirds of the way to the floor for 8 more breaths. Inhale, lift the legs back up, and take the arms out from under the body. Exhale, hugging in the knees.

19. Bridge (Setu Bandhasana)

Lying on the back with the arms alongside the body, place the feet on the floor hip-width apart and parallel, comfortably close to the body (a). Inhale, take the arms back overhead, and lift the hips, grounding through the soles of the feet and lifting the chest toward the chin (b). Exhale, lower the hips to the floor, and take the arms back down from overhead. Repeat the breaths and movements four times. Then stay lifted in bridge for 6 more breaths; inhale, expanding through the chest, and exhale, letting the belly drop in toward the spine.

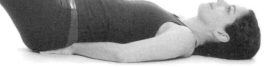

a

b

20. Supported Bridge Legs to Sky (Viparitakarani)

Remain lifted in bridge with the arms along the sides and place a block, horizontally long, under the sacrum. Lift up one leg and then the other so that both legs are extended up with the feet flexed. Stay in viparitakarani for 10 breaths. Then bring both feet back to the floor, remove the block, and lower the hips.

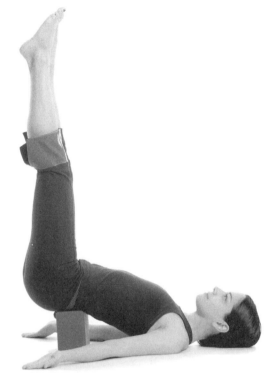

21. Lying Twist With Arm Variations (Jathara Parivrtti)

Hug both knees into the chest. Inhale, extending the arms out to the sides, and exhale, twisting to the right and lowering both knees to the floor. Inhale, lifting the legs back to center, and exhale, twisting to the left *(a)*. Repeat the breathing and movements two times to each side. Then stay in the twist to the left and inhale with the arms open wide. Exhale and take the right hand over and slightly beyond the left hand *(b)*, extending through the shoulder. Inhale and open the right arm again. Repeat the breaths and movements four times and then stay in the twist with the arms open for 6 breaths. Inhale and lift the legs to center. Exhale, twisting to the right, repeat the arm movements four times, and stay for 6 breaths on the other side. Then inhale, lift the legs to center, and hug in the knees.

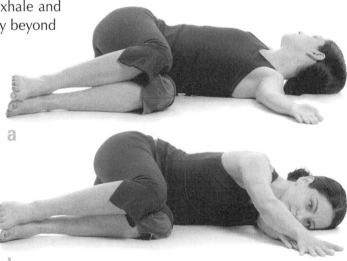

a

b

22. Knees to Chest (Apanasana)

Lying on the back with feet off the floor, place one hand on each knee, fingers pointed toward the toes *(a)*. Inhale, extend the arms, and push the knees forward, keeping the feet off the floor. Exhale and hug the knees in deeply, keeping the head on the floor and drawing the belly in toward the spine *(b)*. Repeat the breath and movement eight times.

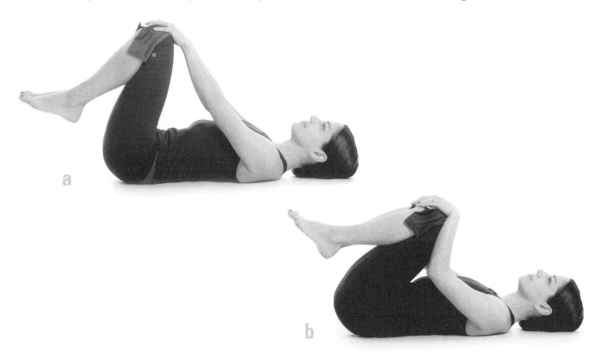

23. Lying Hip Opener

Lying on the back with legs bent and the feet on the floor at hip-width distance, place the left ankle on the top of the right thigh and drop the left knee out to the side to open the left hip. Take the right arm around the outside of the right leg and the left arm between the legs, to interlace the fingers on the top of the right shin. Stay for 8 breaths. Then exhale, drawing the legs in toward the body while keeping the head relaxed to the floor, and inhale, easing up slightly. Release the hands and legs and repeat the pose on the other side.

24. Head-to-Knee Open Twist Forward Bend (Janu Sirsasana)

Sit upright and extend the right leg forward. Place the sole of the left foot to the inside of the right thigh, with the left knee out to the side. Place a blanket under the left knee for support and bend the right leg as much as needed. Hold the inside of the right foot with the right hand and place the left hand to the sacrum at the center of the back *(a)*. Inhale, lengthen the spine, and lift through the chest. Exhale and twist, opening to the left. Inhale, lifting through the chest and leaning back slightly; hold for 6 breaths. Inhale, rotate the hips forward, and take the left hand to meet the right hand over the top of the right foot. Exhale, deepen into the forward bend, and lower the head toward the right knee *(b)*. Stay in the janu sirsasana forward bend for 6 more breaths. Then inhale, expanding through the back of the ribs, and exhale, deepening the forward bend and drawing the belly in toward the spine. Inhale and lift back up, taking the arms overhead, and exhale, relaxing the arms down. Switch legs and repeat both variations of the pose on the other side.

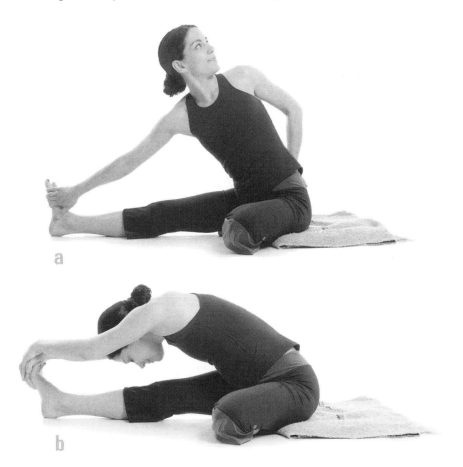

a

b

25. Cobbler's Pose (Baddha Konasana)

Sitting upright on the blanket, bring the soles of the feet together in front of the body, close to the groin. Use the hands to open the feet like a book and externally rotate the hips open *(a)*. Holding the feet, inhale, straighten the arms, and lengthen the spine, lowering the chin to the chest in jalandhara bandha. Stay for 6 breaths, adding a slight pause between the breaths. On the sixth exhalation, round the spine over the legs and extend the arms in front of the body for 6 more breaths *(b)*. Then walk the arms back and inhale, lifting back up again.

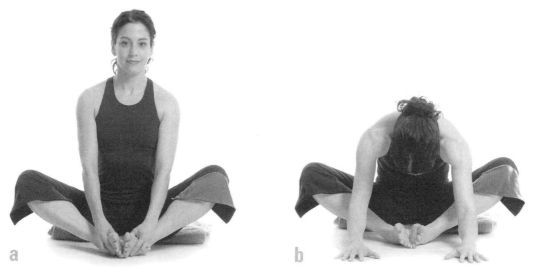

a   b

26. Tabletop

Sitting up, bring the feet flat to the floor and the palms to the floor behind the body, with the fingers facing inward. Inhale and lift the hips, grounding through the feet, lifting the chest, and lowering the head back. If you have neck discomfort, keep the chin lowered toward the chest in jalandhara bandha. Exhale, lower the hips again, and relax the chin to the chest. Repeat the breathing and movements four times and then stay in the tabletop pose for 6 more breaths. Then exhale, lower the hips, and bring the chin to the chest.

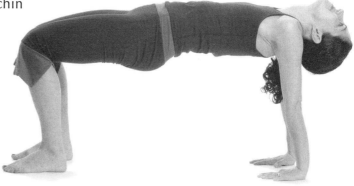

27. Seated Forward Bend With Leg Support (Pascimatanasana)

Extend both legs forward, bending the legs as needed and perhaps even placing a rolled blanket or bolster under the knees. Inhale, lifting the arms overhead *(a)*, and exhale, bending over the legs, placing the hands over the front of the top of the feet, and relaxing the neck completely *(b)*. Stay over the legs and inhale, lifting only the head, and then exhale, releasing it forward again. Repeat this breathing and movement four times to initiate an upper-back stretch and then stay in the forward bend with the neck relaxed for 6 more breaths. Inhale and lift back up, taking the arms overhead, and exhale, relaxing the arms down at the sides.

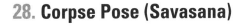

28. Corpse Pose (Savasana)

Lie on the back with the arms at the sides and the palms facing up and extend both legs long, keeping the blanket or bolster under the knees if you used it in the last asana. Let go of the breath and of any tension in the body. Allow the thoughts to come and go freely without letting them take you out of the present moment and the sensation of natural breathing.

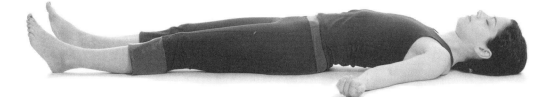

Light 50- to 60-Minute Workout

29. Seated Ocean Breathing (Ujjayi Pranayama)

After a few minutes in savasana, roll over to one side and then gradually come to a seated cross-legged position, sitting on a blanket or padding of some kind for support and comfort. Place the hands on the knees with the palms facing up, the index finger and thumb touching, and the other fingers extended. Close the eyes to bring the focus inward and using ujjayi, or ocean breathing, begin to lengthen the inhalation and deepen the exhalation over the next 4 breaths, gradually finding the boundaries of the breath length. Then for 10 more breaths maintain the long, smooth, steady breathing, adding a slight pause between the inhalation and the exhalation and being mindful of each part of the breath as you experience it. Release the pauses between the breaths and let the inhalation flow into the exhalation for 4 more breaths as a gradual release to natural breathing. Then take a few moments to sit quietly and fully appreciate your peace of mind.

30. Hand-to-the-Heart Invocation

Sit in a cross-legged position. Take the palms together at the heart and close the eyes. Inhale and lift the arms up the sides for the palms to meet overhead. Exhale and bring the palms together down to the heart. Repeat the breathing and movements three times to bring a heartfelt sense of openness and receptivity to the start of the day.

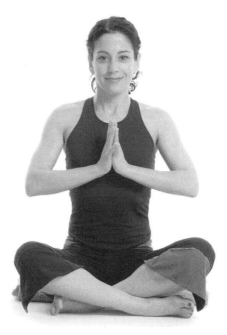

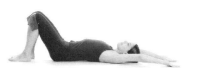

**Breathing Preparations
Lying Arm Movements**

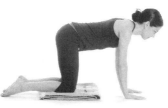

One Knee to the Chest

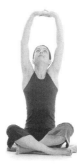

Seated Arm Stretch

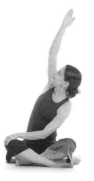

Seated Side Bend

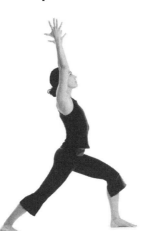

**Cat Vinyasa
Repeat 6 times**

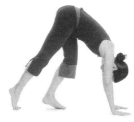

Transition to Standing

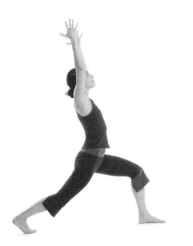

Standing Lunge

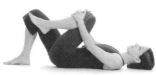

Warrior

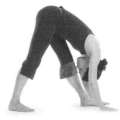

**One-Sided Standing
Forward Bend**

Light 50- to 60-Minute Workout Guide

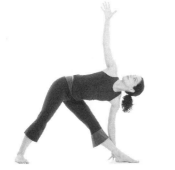

Triangle

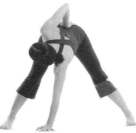

Triangle Twist

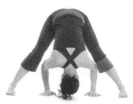

Standing Split Forward Bend

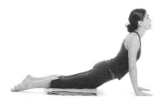

**Kneeling Upward-Facing
Dog Vinyasa
Repeat 6 times**

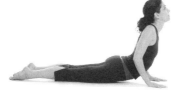

Cobra

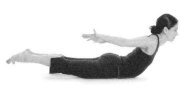

Locust

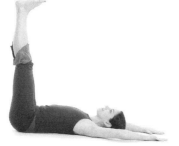

Lying on Back Legs to Sky

Leg Lifts

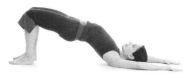

Bridge

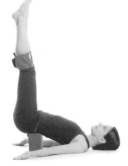

Supported Bridge Legs to Sky

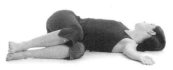

**Lying Twist
With Arm Variations**

Knees to Chest

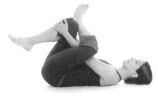

Lying Hip Opener

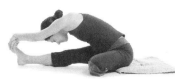

**Head-to-Knee Open Twist
Forward Bend**

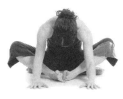

Cobbler's Pose

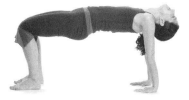

Tabletop

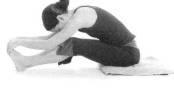

**Seated Forward Bend
With Leg Support**

Corpse Pose

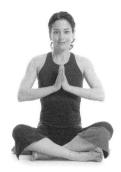

**Seated Ocean Breathing
See page 88**

Hand-to-the-Heart Invocation

5

Moderate Practice

The moderate practices constitute what I'd consider the middle-of-the-road approach to yoga asanas. For a beginner many of the asanas and vinyasas I present as moderate practices will be quite challenging, and perhaps something to work toward as you progress and become proficient though regular practice. For many, and I happily include myself in this category, these practices form a very sustainable foundation for regular practice for the rest of our lives, even for those of us without prohibitive physical considerations who have years of experience in yoga practice. The asanas, vinyasas, and breathing techniques presented as moderate practices are engaging without being overly strenuous and potentially overtaxing. Yoga practice is something that we can continue throughout the many phases and stages of life. These moderate practices should serve as a means in which to move through these phases and stages with regularity, continuity, and grace.

Moderate 15- to 20-Minute Workout

The moderate 20-minute practice is a wonderful minimal morning yoga workout for the committed yogi in a rush. For those days when you are short on time but in need of a basic workout to engage and lengthen the muscles of the body, clear the mind, and energize the spirit before getting out the door, this practice hits the spot.

1. Breathing Preparations

Stand at the front of the mat with the feet about hip-width apart and parallel, the arms at the side, and the gaze forward. Bring your awareness to the breath and begin to lengthen the inhalation and deepen the exhalation using ujjayi, or ocean breathing through the nose, for 6 breaths.

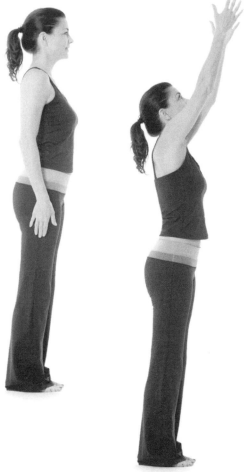

2. Mountain (Tadasana)

In the same standing position, inhale and lift the arms up the sides and overhead, keeping the hands separate and parallel, while gazing up. Start the exhalation and lower the arms down to the sides, lowering the chin down toward the chest. Repeat four times.

3. Standing Forward Bend (Uttanasana)

Inhale, lifting the arms above the head, and exhale, bending over the legs and lowering the hands to the floor. Relax the neck completely and bend the knees as much as needed. Inhale and lift up, taking the arms up the sides to overhead and gazing up slightly. Repeat the breaths and movements up and down four times. Then stay in the forward bend for 6 breaths; inhale, expanding through the back of the body, and exhale, deepening the forward bend. Inhale again and lift back up, taking the arms above the head, and exhale as you lower the arms down along the sides and bring the chin toward the chest.

4. Warrior (Virabhadrasana)

With the arms at the sides, stand in a long split with the right foot forward and the left foot back. The hips, shoulders, and right foot face forward, and the left foot is at a 45-degree angle in the same direction. Inhale, bend the front knee, and lift the arms up the sides and overhead, with the palms separate and facing one another, while looking up slightly *(a)*. Exhale, keep the knee bent, and bend over the right leg, placing the hands on either side of the front foot *(b)*, or on blocks if needed, and relaxing the neck. Ground energy through both feet and inhale, lifting back up and taking the arms up the sides to overhead again. Repeat the breaths and movements four times and then hold the warrior pose for 6 breaths. Exhale, bend over the right leg, and take the hands to the floor (or to blocks) at either side of the right foot, relaxing the neck completely.

a

b

5. One-Sided Standing Forward Bend (Parsva Uttanasana)

Start with the hands on the floor or on blocks at either side of the right foot. Inhale, lengthen the spine, lift the chest, and rotate the hips forward. Exhale and straighten the right leg, drawing the right hip back. Stay in the bend for 6 breaths, grounding through both feet; inhale, expanding through the back of the body and exhale, deepening the forward bend. Then inhale and lift upright, taking the arms up the sides to overhead and keeping the chin toward the chest. Exhale, lower the arms, switch legs, and repeat both this pose and the previous warrior sequence on the other side.

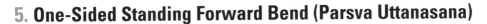

6. Triangle (Trikonasana)

Keep the same foot position as for the previous vinyasa with the left foot forward and the right foot back. Open the shoulders to the side. Inhale and lift the arms out, reaching through the hands. Extend forward and exhale, placing the left hand on the left shin and reaching the right hand up. The left (bottom) hand should be on the shin high enough for the front of the body to stay open. Straighten the legs, with an unlocked left knee. Inhale, ground through the feet, look up, and reach through the right hand with palm open and fingers spread wide *(a)*. Exhale, lower the right arm behind the back, and turn the head to look down at the left foot, keeping the left arm straight *(b)*. Inhale, extend the right arm up again, and repeat the arm movements four times. Then hold the triangle, with the arm extended, for 6 more breaths. Inhale, lifting back up to stand and reaching through the arms, and exhale, lowering the arms to relax. Pivot the feet in the other direction and repeat triangle on the other side.

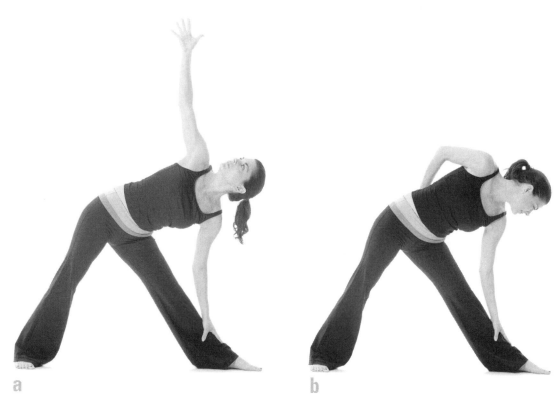

a   b

7. Standing Split Forward Bend (Prasarita Uttanasana)

In a standing split, keep the feet parallel and inhale, extending the arms out to the sides and spreading the palms and fingers wide *(a)*. Exhale and bend over the legs, placing the hands on the floor between the feet *(b)*. Stay over the legs in the forward bend for 6 breaths; inhale, lengthening the spine, and exhale, deepening the forward bend. Relax the neck and bend the knees slightly if needed. Then inhale, lift back upright, and extend the arms out with the palms and fingers open wide. Exhale, taking the palms to meet together at the heart.

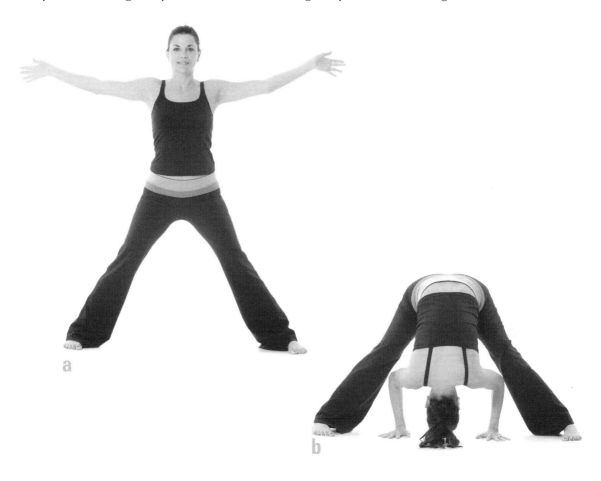

a

b

8. Kneeling Sun Salutation

Come over the hands and knees with the hands in line with the shoulders. Perform kneeling sun salutation as it's described on pages 34–36 in chapter 3. Repeat sequence six times.

Moderate 15- to 20-Minute Workout

9. Transition to Prone Postures

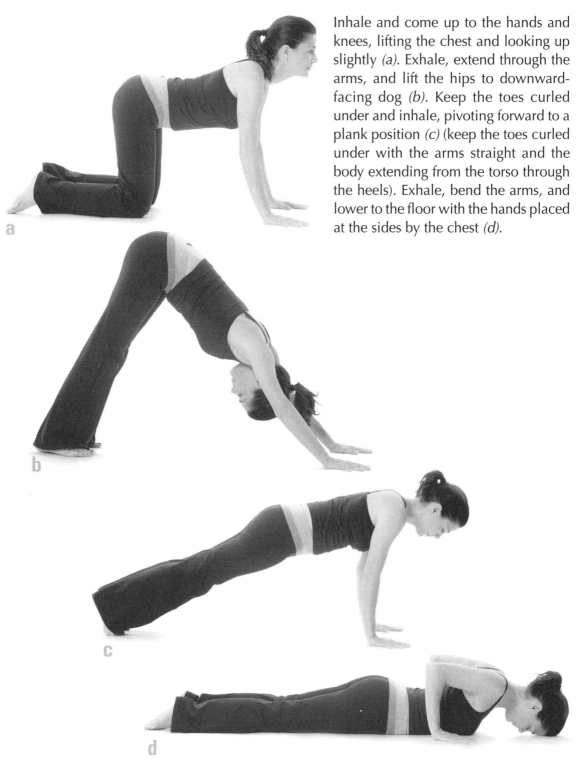

Inhale and come up to the hands and knees, lifting the chest and looking up slightly *(a)*. Exhale, extend through the arms, and lift the hips to downward-facing dog *(b)*. Keep the toes curled under and inhale, pivoting forward to a plank position *(c)* (keep the toes curled under with the arms straight and the body extending from the torso through the heels). Exhale, bend the arms, and lower to the floor with the hands placed at the sides by the chest *(d)*.

10. Cobra (Bhujangasana)

Lie on the front of the body with forehead to the floor and hands placed by the ribs. Inhale, pressing into the hands lightly, and lift the head, neck, and chest up into cobra. Exhale and lower the head, neck, and chest back down. Repeat the breath and movements four times and then stay in the cobra for 6 breaths. Exhale, staying lifted, and let the belly press into the floor. Inhale, lifting through the chest, and then exhale and relax back to the floor.

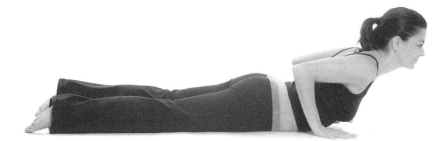

11. Bow (Dhanurasana)

Lying on the front of the body, bend the knees and reach back to hold the ankles. Flex the feet slightly and spread the toes, keeping the legs relatively close but not jammed together. Inhale and lift the head, neck, chest, feet, and legs, allowing the shoulders to rotate back and opening through the chest. Stay in the bow for 8 breaths. Exhale, lower back down, release the feet, and relax.

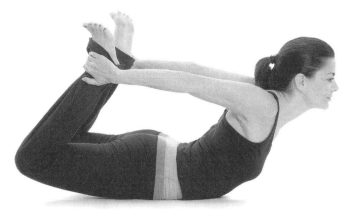

12. Child's Pose (Balasana) to Cat

Come to child's pose with the hips to the heels, the arms extended in front of the body, and the forehead relaxed to the floor *(a)*. Inhale and come up to the hands and knees, lifting the chest and looking up slightly *(b)*. Exhale, round the spine, and come back to child's pose. Repeat the breathing and movements six times, releasing any tension in the lower back from cobra and bow.

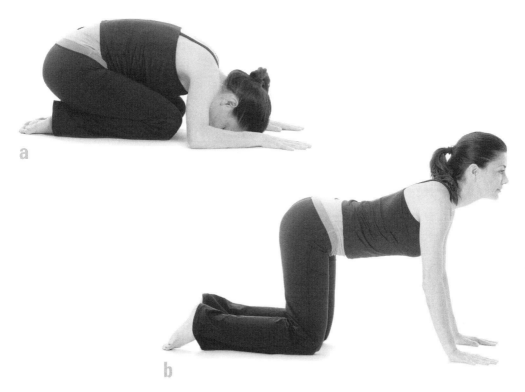

13. Seated Twist (Ardha Matsyendrasana)

Take a seated position with both legs extended forward. Place the right foot to the outside of the left thigh, leaving the left leg long. Place the left arm along the outside of the right thigh and place the right hand, lifted lightly on the fingertips, on the floor behind the body. Soften the gaze to take the focus inward. Inhale, lifting and lengthening the spine, and exhale, engaging the twist to the right, drawing the belly in and up, and turning the head in the same direction. Be mindful not to strain the spine by forcing through the arms and shoulders. Stay in the twist for 6 breaths and then release; repeat the twist to the left.

14. Seated Mindful Breathing

Sit in a cross-legged seated position with the hands at the knees, palms facing up. Take 10 steady, smooth, long, mindful breaths with the eyes closed. Then open the eyes and move into the start of your day with rejuvenated energy.

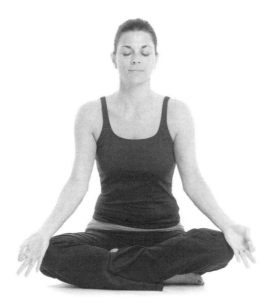

Moderate 15- to 20-Minute Workout Guide

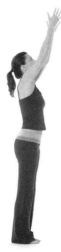
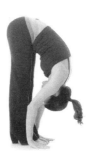
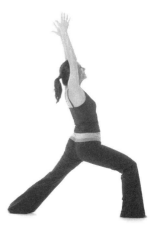

Breathing Preparations Mountain

Standing Forward Bend

Warrior

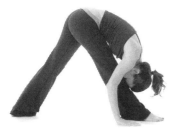
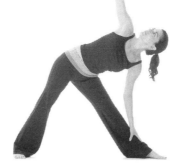
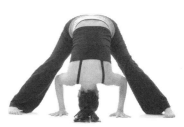

One-Sided Standing Forward Bend

Triangle

Standing Split Forward Bend

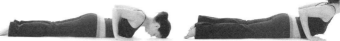

Kneeling Sun Salutation See pages 35–36

Transition to Prone Postures

Cobra

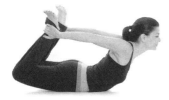

Bow

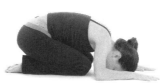

Child's Pose to Cat

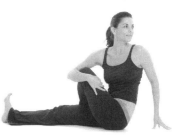

Seated Twist

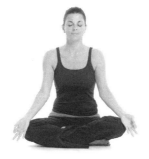

Seated Mindful Breathing

Moderate 30- to 40-Minute Workout

This morning yoga workout is what I consider to be the middle path of the morning yoga workouts presented in the book. In 40 minutes we can work deeply but with a pace and an intensity level that is satisfyingly energetic without being overly exertive or draining.

1. Breathing Preparations

Stand at the front of the mat with the feet together, the arms at the sides, and the gaze forward. Bring your awareness to the breath and begin to lengthen the inhalation and deepen the exhalation using ujjayi, or ocean breathing through the nose, for 6 breaths.

2. Mountain (Tadasana)

In the same standing position, inhale and lift the arms up the sides and overhead, keeping the hands separate to leave space for the shoulders, while gazing up. Start the exhalation, lower the arms down the sides, and lower the chin down toward the chest. Repeat four times.

3. Standing Forward Bend (Uttanasana)

Inhale, lifting the arms above the head, and exhale, bending over the legs and lowering the hands to the floor. Relax the neck completely and bend the knees as much as needed. Inhale and lift up, taking the arms up the sides and overhead and gazing up slightly. Repeat the breaths and movements up and down four times. Then stay in the forward bend for 6 breaths; inhale, expanding through the back of the body, and exhale, deepening the forward bend. Inhale again, lifting back up and taking the arms above the head, and exhale as you lower the arms down along the sides and bring the chin toward the chest.

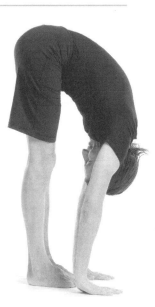

4. Chair (Utkatasana)

Start with the feet hip-width apart and parallel. Inhale, lift the arms above the head with hands separate and palms facing each other, and gaze forward with the chin toward the chest *(a)*. Exhale, bend the knees, and lower the hips level with the knees, keeping the heels on the floor if possible or placing a rolled blanket under the heels if needed *(b)*. Inhale, straightening the legs, and exhale, bending the knees and lowering the hips. Repeat the breaths and movements six times and then stay in utkatasana pose for 6 breaths. Then inhale, lifting back to stand, and exhale, lowering the arms down the sides.

a

b

5. Sun Salutation A

Perform sun salutation A as it's described on pages 36–38 in chapter 3. Repeat sequence six times.

6. Warrior I (Virabhadrasana I) to One-Sided Standing Forward Bend (Parsva Uttanasana)

Step into a long split with the right leg forward and the left leg back. Rotate the hips and shoulders forward, and turn the left foot outward at a 45-degree angle in the same direction. Inhale, look up slightly, bend the right knee, and lift the arms up the sides to overhead, with the palms facing each other, separate and parallel *(a)*. Exhale, straighten the right leg, and take the arms down the sides, placing the palms at either side of the right foot *(b)*. Again inhale, bend the right knee, and take the arms up the sides, lifting to warrior. Repeat the breathing and movements four times. Then stay in warrior for 6 breaths and in the forward bend over the right leg for 6 more. Inhale, lifting back to warrior once more, and exhale, relaxing the arms back down the sides, straightening the front leg, and lowering the chin to the chest. Switch legs and repeat vinyasa on the other side.

a

b

7. Warrior II (Virabhadrasana II)

Come into the same split stance as for warrior I, starting with the left leg forward and the right leg back. Open the shoulders to the right, keeping the hips rotated forward *(a)*. Inhale, lift the arms with the palms facing down, extending out through the fingers, and then exhale, bending the left knee deeply *(b)*. Your stance should be long enough that the bent left knee does not go beyond the left ankle. Look first over the right hand, grounding energy through the right leg and reaching through both arms. Then turn the head and look over the left hand. Stay in the warrior II pose for 6 breaths. Inhale, straightening the left leg, and exhale, relaxing the arms down at the sides. Pivot the feet and repeat the same warrior II on the other side.

a

b

8. Triangle (Trikonasana)

With right leg forward and left leg back in the same split stance as for warrior II just completed, open the shoulders to the left side *(a)*. Inhale and lift the arms out, reaching through the hands. Exhale, lowering the right hand to the right shin, or to the outside of the right foot, and reaching the left hand up. Straighten legs, with an unlocked right knee. Inhale, grounding through the feet, look up, and reach through the top hand with palm open and fingers spread wide *(b)*. Exhale, lower the left arm behind the back, and turn the head to look down at the right foot, keeping the right arm straight and the front of the body open *(c)*. Inhale, extend the left arm up again, and repeat the arm movements for 4 breaths. Then hold trikonasana for 6 breaths. Inhale, lifting back up to stand and reaching through the arms, and exhale, lowering the arms to the sides to relax. Pivot the feet in the other direction and repeat triangle on the other side.

a

b

c

9. Extended Side Angle (Utthita Parsva Konasana)

In the same split stance as for triangle, inhale and reach the arms out to the sides. Exhale, bend the left knee, and place the left hand at the inside of the left shin, or on a block placed on the outside of the left foot, and the right hand on the right hip. Rotate the left thigh and hip open and back and, grounding through the right leg, reach the right arm forward overhead. Draw the right shoulder back in its socket slightly and gaze either directly up into the armpit or to the side. Stay in utthita parsva konasana pose for 6 breaths. Then exhale, take the right hand back to the right hip, and look down at the left foot. Inhale and reach both arms out, lifting upright and straightening the left leg. Exhale and relax the arms down at the sides. Pivot the feet and repeat extended angle pose in the other direction.

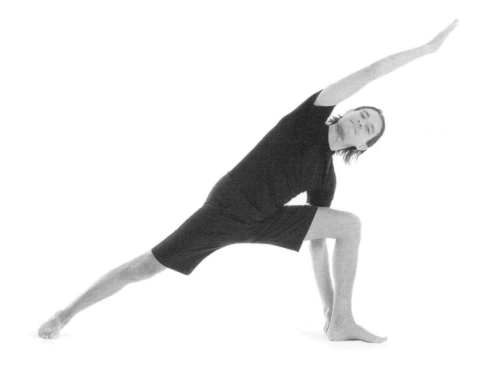

10. Triangle Twist (Parivrtti Trikonasana)

Come into a wide split with the feet parallel and the arms at the sides. Inhale and reach the arms out to the sides *(a)*. Exhale and twist through the torso to the right, placing the left hand at the floor next to the right foot, extending the right hand with the palm wide, and looking up. Inhale, reach through both arms, and lift back to center. Exhale and twist to the left, placing the right hand next to the left foot, extending the right hand up with the palm wide, and looking up *(b)*. Repeat twist four times to each side. On the fourth repetition on each side, stay in the twist for 6 breaths; exhale, deepening the twist, and inhale, easing up slightly to lengthen the spine. Then inhale, lifting back to cent:er and reaching through both arms, and exhale, relaxing the arms to the sides.

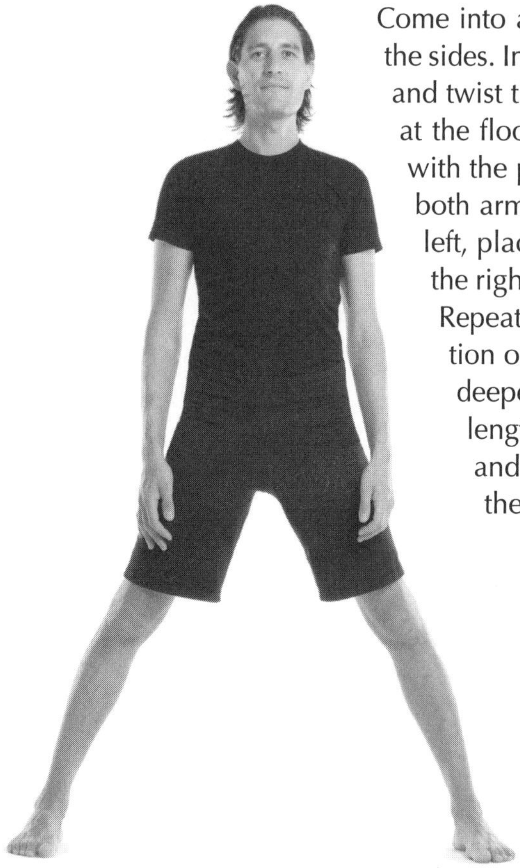

a

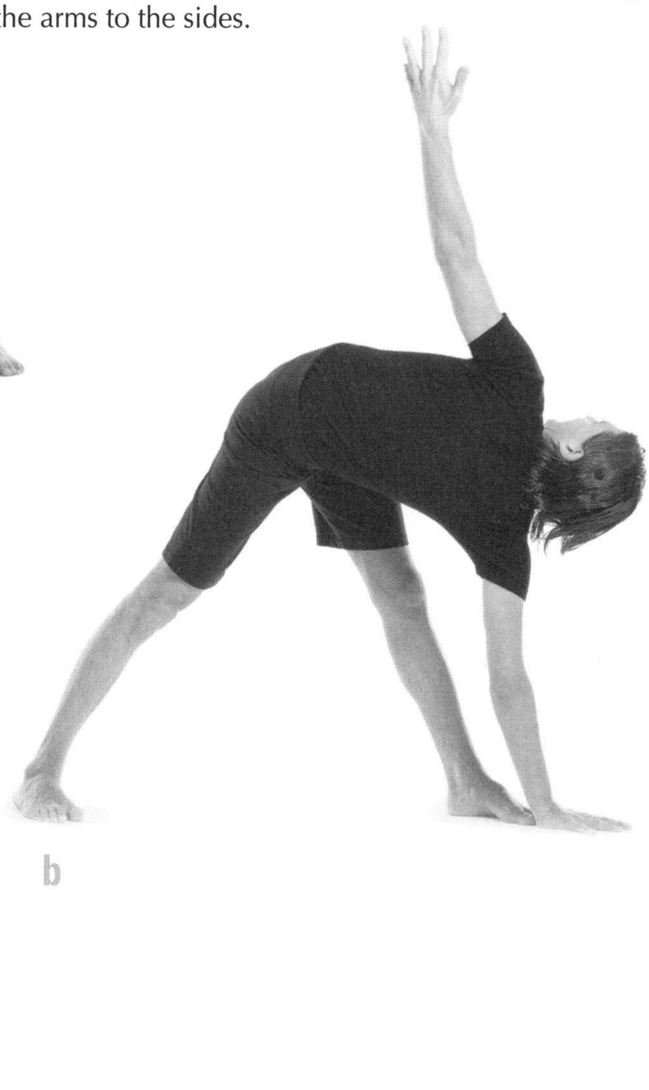

b

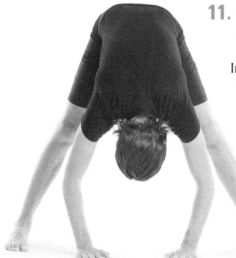

11. Standing Split Forward Bend (Prasarita Uttanasana)

In a standing split, take the feet parallel and inhale, extending the arms out to the sides and spreading the palms and fingers wide. Exhale and bend over the legs, placing the hands on the floor between the feet. Stay over the legs in the forward bend for 6 breaths. Then inhale, lengthening the spine, and exhale, deepening the forward bend. Relax the neck and bend the knees slightly if needed. Inhale, come back upright, and extend the arms out with the palms and fingers open wide. Exhale, bringing the palms to meet at the heart.

12. Tree Pose (Vrksasana)

Come to stand at the front of the mat with the feet together and the arms at the sides. Place the right hand on the right hip. With the left arm, guide the sole of the left foot up to the inside of the right thigh and open the left hip. Gaze at a point in front of you and bring the palms together at the heart *(a)*. Ground down through the straight right leg but keep the right knee unlocked, and extend upward through the torso. Inhale, lift the palms together up above the head, and then separate and open the arms and spread the fingers wide *(b)*. Stay in tree pose for 6 breaths. Exhale, bringing the palms together down to the heart and releasing the left foot down. Repeat tree pose on the other side.

a

b

Moderate 30- to 40-Minute Workout

13. Lying on Back Legs to Sky (Urdva Prasarita Padasana)

Lie on the back and hug the knees to the chest, with one hand on each knee *(a)*. Inhale, extend the legs up, and flex the feet as you take the arms back overhead, wide enough apart that the shoulders can comfortably connect to the floor *(b)*. Exhale and hug the knees to the chest again. Repeat the breath and movement six times. Then stay for 6 breaths with the legs extended and the arms back over the head. On the last exhalation, hug in the knees and relax.

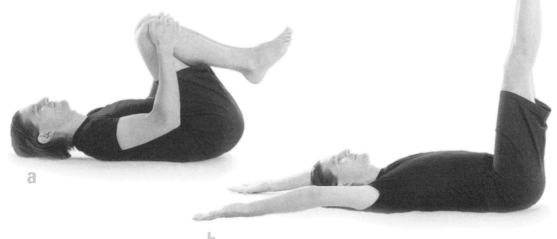

14. Leg Lifts (Urdva Padasana)

Lying on the back, take the arms slightly underneath the body with the palms face down and bend the knees to the chest. Inhale, extend the legs up, and flex the feet. Exhale and hold. Then inhale, lowering the legs about two-thirds of the way to the floor, and exhale, lifting up the legs again and bending the knees slightly at the top of the pose to ease lower-back tension. Repeat the breaths and movements six times and then hold the pose with the legs about two-thirds of the way to the floor for 8 more breaths. Inhale, lift the legs back up, and take the arms out from under the body. Exhale, hugging in the knees.

15. Boat (Navasana)

Rock up to sit, bend the knees, and bring the feet flat to the floor. Inhale, extending the arms out in front of the body *(a)*, and exhale, lifting the feet off the floor. Inhale and straighten the legs, extending through the arms and rounding the back slightly *(b)*; stay for in boat for 6 breaths. To release the pose, inhale, lowering the legs to the floor and lifting the arms above the head, and then exhale, lowering the arms down to the sides.

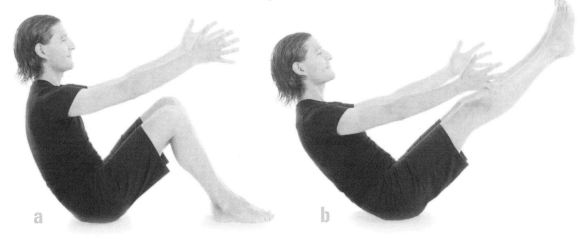

a   b

16. Seated Forward Bend (Pascimatanasana)

Remain seated with both legs extended forward and the hands at the hips, sitting on a blanket if needed. Inhale, lifting the arms overhead *(a)*, and exhale, bending over the legs, placing the hands over the top of the feet, and relaxing the neck *(b)*. Allow the natural curvature of the spine to occur and bend the knees if needed to allow the hips to rotate and the lower abdomen to connect with the upper thighs. Inhale and lift back up, taking the arms overhead, and exhale, bending over the legs again. Repeat the breathing and movements four times and then stay in the forward bend for 6 more breaths; inhale, expanding through the back of the ribs, and exhale, deepening the forward bend and drawing the belly in and up. Then inhale and lift back up, taking the arms overhead, and exhale, relaxing the arms down to the sides.

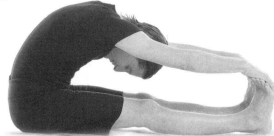

a   b

17. Bridge (Setu Bandhasana)

Lie on the back with the knees bent, the feet parallel at hip-width distance, and the arms alongside the body *(a)*. Inhale, take the arms back overhead, and lift the hips *(b)*. Exhale, bring the arms back down alongside the body, and lower the hips. Repeat the breaths and movements four times and then stay in bridge for 6 breaths; inhale, opening through the chest and exhale, letting the belly drop in toward the spine. Then to release the bridge, exhale and take the arms back down alongside the body, and lower the hips.

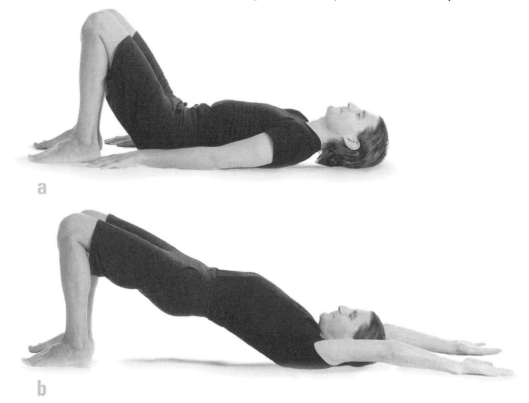

a

b

18. Shoulder Stand (Sarvangasana) to Plow (Halasana)

Lie on the back with the knees bent, the feet flat, and the arms alongside the body, palms facing down. Feel free to place a blanket under the shoulder and upper back, with the neck off the floor for extra support. Exhale and roll back onto the shoulders, bringing the feet to the floor behind the head *(a)*. With the arms in comfortably close, bend the elbows and place the hands flat on the back. Inhale and lift the legs up to the ceiling *(b)*. Point through the feet and curl back the toes so that both the front and back of the legs are actively lifting in the shoulder stand. Stay lifted for 12 breaths. Then exhale and lower the right knee to the chest, keeping the left leg lifted *(c)*. Inhale, lifting the right leg up, and exhale, lowering the left knee to the chest. Repeat the breathing and movements, alternating two times on each side. Then exhale, lowering both knees to the chest, and inhale, lifting the legs back up; repeat four times. Exhale, lowering both feet to the floor behind the head and the arms to the floor beside the body. Stay in plow pose, or halasana, for 6 breaths. Then inhale, roll down to lie on the back, and exhale to rest.

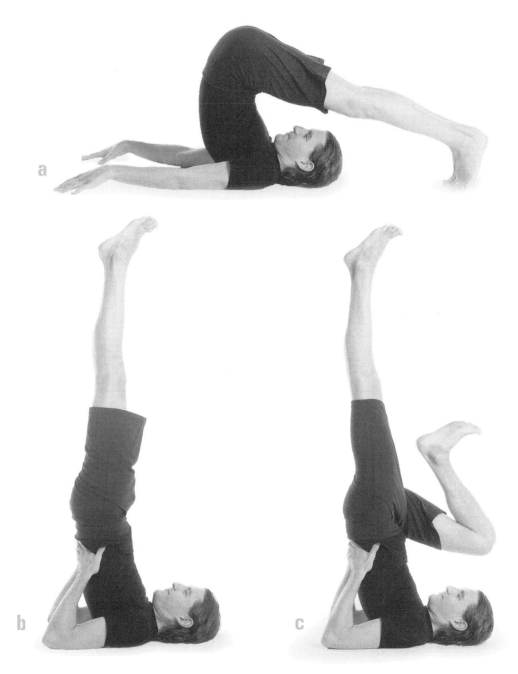

Moderate 30- to 40-Minute Workout

19. Corpse Pose (Savasana)

Lie on the back and extend both legs long, with the arms at the sides and the palms facing up. Let go of the breath and of any tension in the body. Let the thoughts come and go freely without allowing them to take you out of the present moment and the sensation of natural breathing for a few minutes.

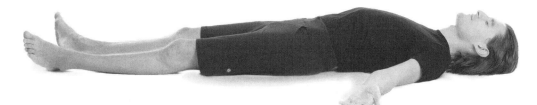

20. Cobra (Bhujangasana)

Roll over onto the front of the body and lie with the forehead to the floor and the hands placed by the ribs. Inhale, pressing into the hands lightly, and lift the head, neck, and chest up into cobra. Exhale and lower the head, neck, and chest back down. Repeat the breaths and movements four times. Then stay in cobra for 6 breaths; exhale, staying lifted and letting the belly press into the floor, and inhale, lifting through the chest. Then exhale and relax back to the floor.

21. Bow (Dhanurasana)

Bend the knees and reach back to hold the ankles. Flex the feet slightly and spread the toes, keeping the legs relatively close but not jammed together. Inhale and lift the head, neck, chest, feet, and legs, allowing the shoulders to rotate back and opening through the chest. Stay in bow for 8 breaths. Exhale, lower back down, release the feet, and relax.

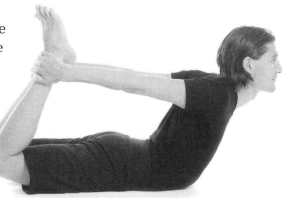

22. Child's Pose (Balasana) to Cat

Come to child's pose with the hips to the heels, the arms extended in front of the body, and the forehead relaxed to the floor *(a)*. Inhale and come up to the hands and knees, lifting the chest and looking up slightly *(b)*. Exhale, round the spine into cat, and come back to child's pose. Repeat the breathing and movement six times, releasing any tension in the lower back from cobra and bow.

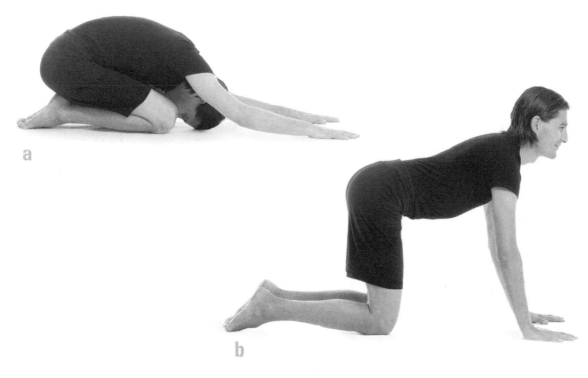

23. Alternate Nostril Breathing (Nadi Sodhana Pranayama)

Take a comfortable seated position. Extend the right hand forward with the palm facing up. Bring the index and the middle fingers into the palm. Bring the right hand to the nose, placing the ring finger on the left nostril and the thumb on the right, just below the bridge of the nose. Take one full breath through both nostrils. Then close off the left nostril completely with the ring finger and inhale through the right. Close both nostrils and hold the breath in, lowering the chin toward the chest. Release the ring finger and exhale through the left nostril. Hold the breath out for a few seconds and then inhale through the left nostril. Close both nostrils, hold the breath in for a few seconds, release the right nostril, and exhale to complete one full round of alternate nostril breathing. Repeat nadi sodhana for six full rounds or 12 breaths, finishing with an exhalation through the right nostril. Then relax the right hand down and breathe freely, taking a few minutes to experience the peaceful, clear state of mind you have cultivated to begin the start of your day.

Moderate 30- to 40-Minute Workout Guide

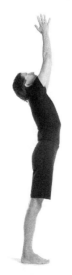

**Breathing Preparations
Mountain**

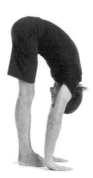

Standing Forward Bend

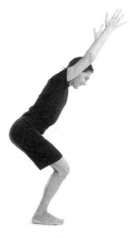

Chair

**Sun Salutation A
See pages 37-38**

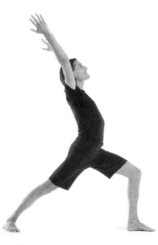

**Warrior I to One-Sided
Standing Forward Bend**

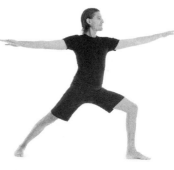

Warrior II

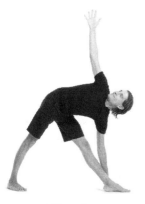

Triangle

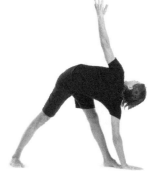

Extended Side Angle

Triangle Twist

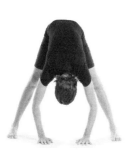

Standing Split Forward Bend

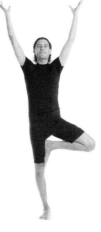

Tree Pose

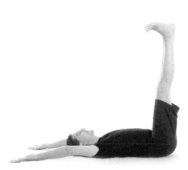

Lying on Back Legs to Sky

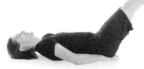

Leg Lifts

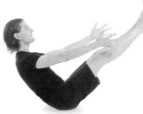

Boat

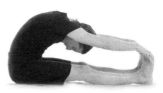

Seated Forward Bend

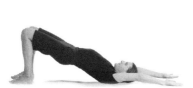

Bridge

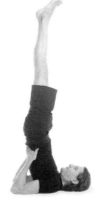

Shoulder Stand to Plow

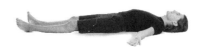

Corpse Pose

Moderate 30- to 40-Minute Workout Guide

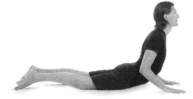

Cobra

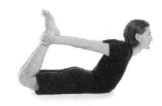

Bow

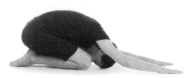

Child's Pose to Cat

Alternate Nostril Breathing
See page 10

A long, unrushed yoga practice right at the start of the day is so satisfying. For days when we have plenty of time on hand, this moderate 60-minute moderate practice is a treat. Building on the moderate 20- and 40-minute practices, we can experience a fuller range of asanas, vinyasas, and breathing exercises to compose a complete moderate practice.

1. Breathing Preparations

Stand at the front of the mat with the feet hip-width apart and parallel, the arms at the sides, and the gaze forward. Bring your awareness to the breath and begin to lengthen the inhalations and deepen the exhalations using ujjayi, or ocean breathing through the nose, for 6 breaths.

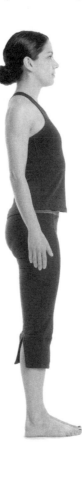

2. Mountain (Tadasana)

In the same standing position, inhale and lift the arms up the sides and overhead, keeping the hands separate to leave space for the shoulders, while gazing up. Start the exhalation and lower the arms down the sides, lowering the chin down toward the chest. Repeat four times.

3. Standing Forward Bend (Uttanasana)

Inhale, lifting the arms above the head, and exhale, bending over the legs and lowering the hands to the floor. Relax the neck completely and bend the knees as much as needed. Inhale and lift up, taking the arms up the sides to overhead and gazing up slightly. Repeat the breaths and movements up and down four times. Then stay in the forward bend for 6 breaths; inhale, expanding through the back of the body, and exhale, deepening the forward bend. Inhale again and lift back up, taking the arms above the head, and exhale as you lower the arms down along the sides and bring the chin toward the chest.

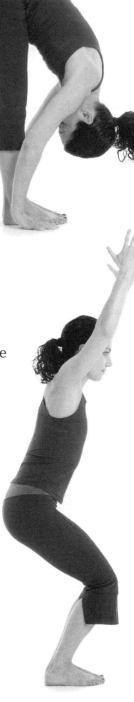

4. Chair (Utkatasana)

Start with the feet hip-width apart and parallel. Inhale, lift the arms above the head with hands separate and palms facing each other, and gaze forward with the chin toward the chest. Exhale, bend the knees, and lower the hips to knee level, keeping the heels on the floor if possible or placing a rolled blanket under the heels if needed. Inhale, straightening the legs, and exhale, bending the knees and lowering the hips. Repeat the breaths and movements six times and then stay in utkatasana pose for 6 breaths. Then inhale, lifting back to stand, and exhale, lowering the arms down the sides.

5. Sun Salutation A

Perform sun salutation A as it's described on pages 36–38 in chapter 3. Repeat sequence six times.

6. Sun Salutation B

Perform sun salutation B as it's described on pages 38–40 in chapter 3. Repeat sequence six times.

7. Warrior II (Virabhadrasana II)

Come into the same split stance as warrior I, starting with the left leg forward and the right leg back. Open the shoulders to the right, keeping the hips rotated forward. Inhale, lift the arms with the palms facing down, extending out through the fingers, and then exhale, bending the left knee deeply. Your stance should be long enough that the bent left knee does not go beyond the left ankle. Look first over the right hand, grounding energy through the right leg and reaching through both arms. Then turn the head and look over the left hand. Stay in warrior II pose for 6 breaths. Inhale, straightening the left leg, and exhale, relaxing the arms down at the sides. Pivot the feet and repeat the same warrior II on the other side.

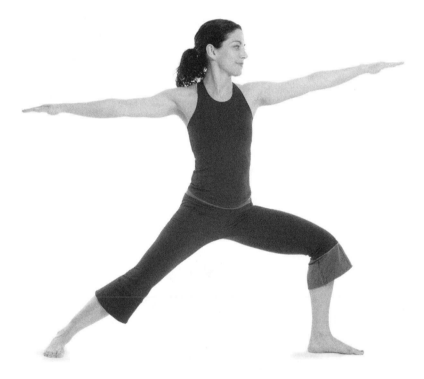

8. Triangle (Trikonasana)

With right leg forward and left leg back in the same split stance as for warrior II, open the shoulders to the left side. Inhale and lift the arms out, reaching through the hands. Exhale, lowering the right hand to the right shin and reaching the left hand up. Straighten legs, with an unlocked right knee. Inhale, grounding through the feet, look up, and reach through the top hand with palm open and fingers spread wide *(a)*. Exhale, lower the left arm behind the back, and turn the head to look down at the right foot, keeping the right arm straight and the front of the body open *(b)*. Inhale, extend the left arm up again, and repeat the arm movements for 4 breaths. Then hold the trikonasana for 6 breaths. Inhale, lifting back up to stand and reaching through the arms, and exhale, lowering the arms to the sides to relax. Pivot the feet in the other direction and repeat triangle on the other side.

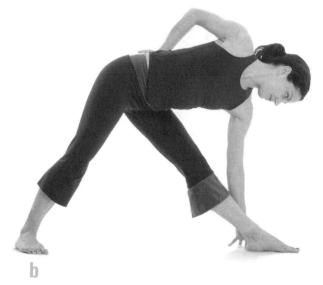

a

b

9. Extended Side Angle (Utthita Parsva Konasana)

In the same split stance as for triangle, inhale and reach the arms out to the sides. Exhale, bend the left knee, and place the left hand at the inside of the left shin, or on a block placed on the outside of the left foot, and the right hand on the right hip. Rotate the left thigh and hip open and back and, grounding through the right leg, reach the right arm forward overhead. Draw the right shoulder back in socket slightly and gaze either directly up into the armpit or to the side. Stay in utthita parsva konasana for 6 breaths. Then exhale, take the right hand back to the right hip, and look down at the left foot. Inhale and reach both arms out, lifting upright and straightening the left leg. Exhale and relax the arms down at the sides. Pivot the feet and repeat extended angle pose in the other direction.

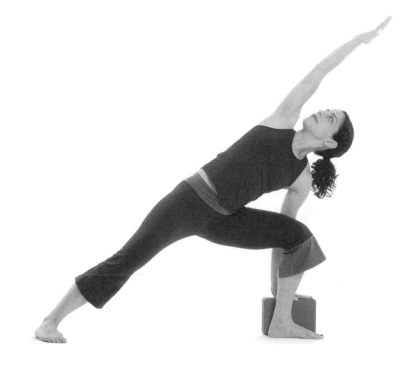

10. Triangle Twist (Parivrtti Trikonasana)

Come into a wide split with the feet parallel and the arms at the sides. Inhale and reach the arms out to the sides *(a)*. Exhale and twist through the torso to the right, placing the left hand at the floor between the feet, extending the right hand with the palm wide, and looking up *(b)*. Inhale, reach through both arms, and lift back to center. Exhale and twist to the left, placing the right hand between the feet, extending the left hand up with the palm wide, and looking up. Repeat breathing and twist four times to each side. On the fourth repetition on each side, stay in the twist for 6 breaths; exhale, deepening the twist, and inhale, easing up slightly to lengthen the spine. Then inhale, lifting back to center and reaching through both arms, and exhale, relaxing the arms to the sides.

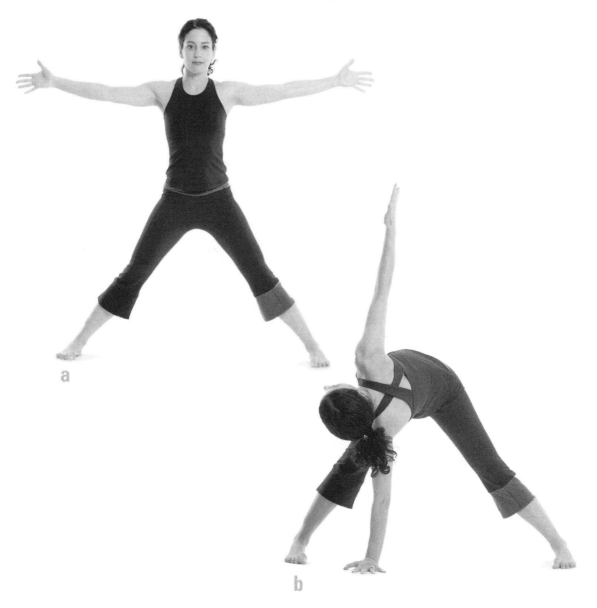

a

b

11. Standing Split Forward Bend (Prasarita Uttanasana)

In a standing split, keep the feet parallel and inhale, extending the arms out to the sides and spreading the palms and fingers wide. Exhale and bend over the legs, placing the hands on the floor between the feet. Stay over the legs in the forward bend for 6 breaths; inhale, lengthening the spine, and exhale, deepening the forward bend. Relax the neck and bend the knees slightly if needed. Then inhale, lift back upright, and extend the arms out with the palms and fingers open wide. Exhale, taking the palms to meet together at the heart.

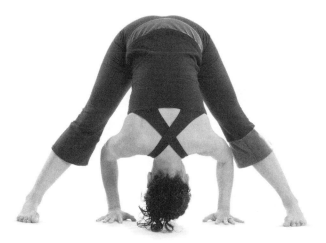

12. Warrior III (Virabhadrasana III)

Stand at the front of the mat, gazing forward, with the feet hip-width apart and the arms at the sides. Inhale and lift the arms out to the sides. Exhale, keeping a long spine, and hinge at the hips to bend forward while you lift the right leg up behind, keeping the foot perpendicular to the floor *(a)*. Keep the left leg straight with an unlocked knee. Inhale and reach the arms forward, with the palms parallel and facing each other *(b)*. Stay in warrior III for 6 breaths. Then inhale and lift back up, lowering the right foot to meet the left and lowering the arms. Exhale, relaxing the arms down at the sides. Repeat the asana on the other side.

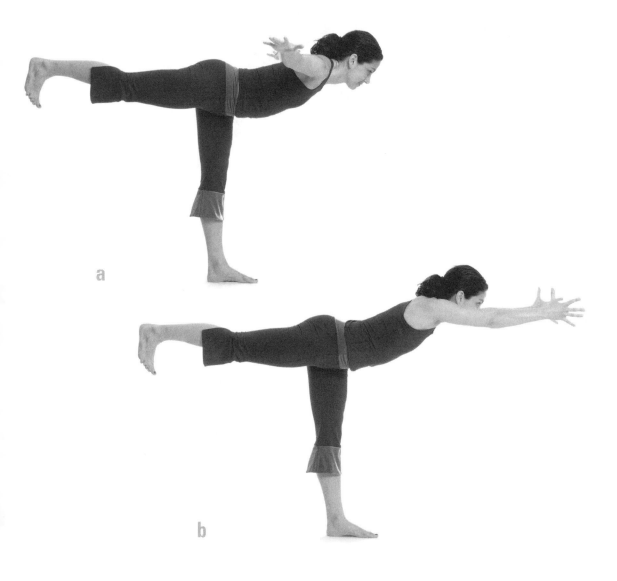

13. Tree Pose (Vrksasana)

Come to stand at the front of the mat with the feet together and the arms at the sides. Place the right hand on the right hip. With the left arm, guide the sole of the left foot up to the inside of the right thigh and open the left hip. Gaze at a point in front of you and bring the palms together at the heart *(a)*. Ground down through the straight right leg but keep the right knee unlocked, and extend upward through the torso. Inhale, lift the palms together up above the head, and then separate the palms and open the arms, spreading the fingers wide *(b)*. Stay in tree pose for 6 breaths. Exhale, bringing the palms together down to the heart and releasing the left foot down. Repeat tree pose on the other side.

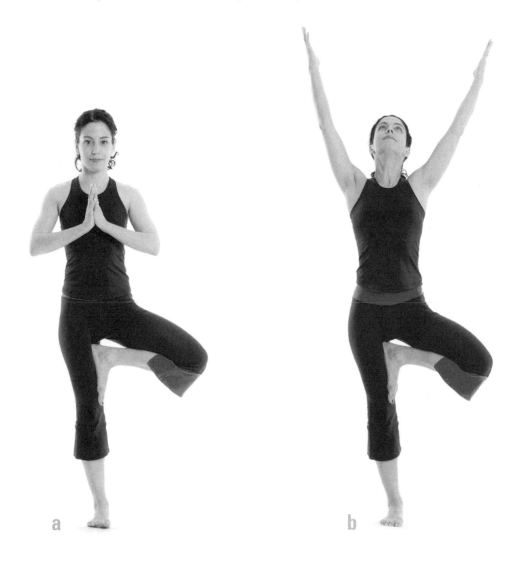

a   b

14. Transition to Cobra (Bhujangasana)

Stand at the front of the mat with the feet parallel and hip-width apart and the arms at the sides. Inhale, gazing up slightly, and lift the arms up the sides for the palms to meet overhead. Exhale, bend over the legs, bringing the arms down the sides, and place the hands on either side of the feet *(a)*. Inhale and stay in the forward bend, lengthening the spine and lifting the chest. Exhale and deepen the forward bend, bringing the palms flat on the floor and bending the knees slightly. Holding the breath out, lightly hop back *(b)* to plank *(c)* (keep the toes curled under and the arms straight with the body extending from the torso through the heels). Keeping the toes curled under, inhale into upward-facing dog *(d)* and then exhale, bending the elbows and lowering to the floor.

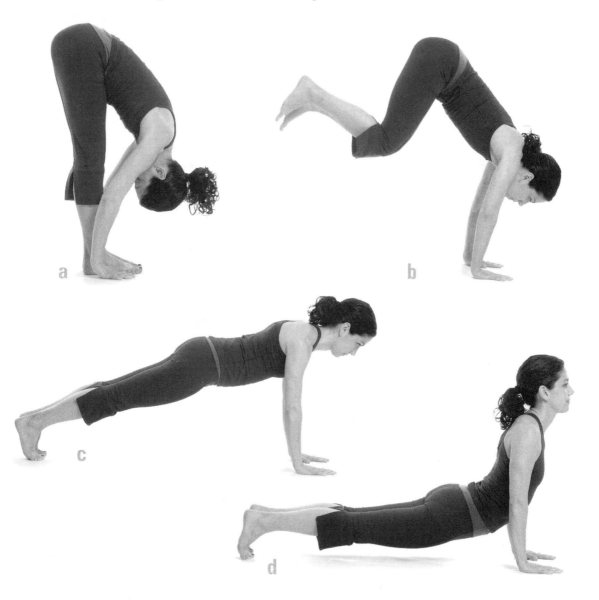

15. Cobra (Bhujangasana)

Lie on the front of the body with the forehead to the floor and the hands placed by the ribs _(a)_. Inhale, pressing into the hands lightly, and lift the head, neck, and chest up into cobra _(b)_. Exhale and lower the head, neck, and chest back down. Repeat the breath and movements four times and then stay in cobra for 6 breaths; exhale, staying lifted and letting the belly press into the floor, and inhale, lifting through the chest. Then exhale and relax back to the floor.

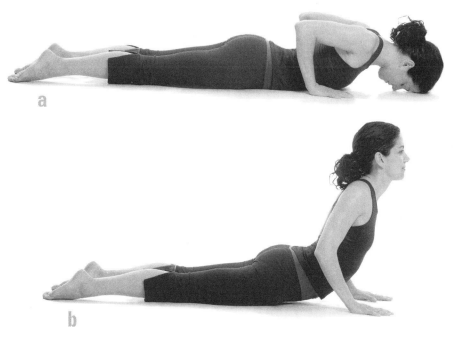

16. Bow (Dhanurasana)

Bend the knees and reach back to hold the ankles. Flex the feet slightly and spread the toes, keeping the legs relatively close but not jammed together. Inhale and lift the head, neck, chest, feet, and legs, allowing the shoulders to rotate back and opening through the chest. Stay in bow for 8 breaths. Exhale, lower back down, release the feet, and relax.

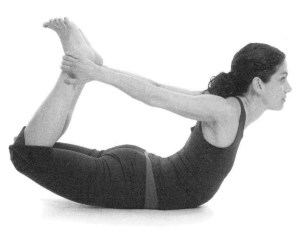

17. Lying on Back Legs to Sky (Urdva Prasarita Padasana)

Lie on the back and hug the knees to the chest, with one hand on each knee *(a)*. Inhale, extend the legs up, and flex the feet as you take the arms back overhead, wide enough apart that the shoulders can comfortably connect to the floor *(b)*. Exhale and hug the knees to the chest again. Repeat the breath and movement six times. Then stay for 6 breaths with the legs extended and the arms back over the head. On the last exhalation, hug in the knees and relax.

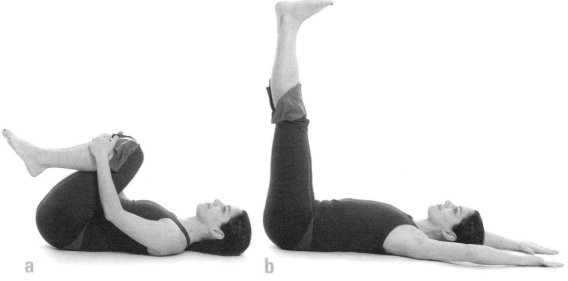

a   b

18. Leg Lifts (Urdva Padasana)

Lying on the back, take the arms slightly underneath the body with the palms face down and bend the knees to the chest. Inhale, extend the legs up, and flex the feet. Exhale and hold. Then inhale, lowering the legs about two-thirds of the way to the floor, and exhale, lifting up the legs again and bending the knees slightly at the top of the pose to ease lower-back tension. Repeat the breaths and movements six times and then hold the pose with the legs about two-thirds of the way to the floor for 8 more breaths. Inhale, lift the legs back up, and take the arms out from under the body. Exhale, hugging in the knees.

19. Boat (Navasana)

Rock up to sit, bend the knees, and bring the feet flat to the floor. Inhale, extending the arms out in front of the body, and exhale, lifting the feet off the floor. Inhale and straighten the legs, extending through the arms and rounding the back slightly; stay for 6 breaths. Then inhale, lowering the legs to the floor and lifting the arms above the head, and exhale, lowering the arms down to the sides.

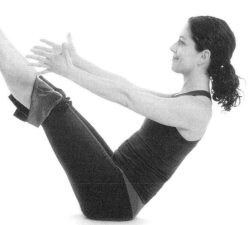

20. Seated Forward Bend (Pascimatanasana)

Remain seated with both legs extended forward and the hands at the hips, sitting on a blanket if needed. Inhale, lifting the arms overhead, and exhale, bending over the legs, placing the hands over the top of the feet, and relaxing the neck. Allow the natural curvature of the spine to occur and bend the knees if needed to allow the hips to rotate and the lower abdomen to connect with the upper thighs. Inhale and lift back up, taking the arms overhead, and exhale, bending over the legs again. Repeat the breathing and movements four times and then stay in the forward bend for 6 more breaths; inhale, expanding through the back of the ribs, and exhale, deepening the forward bend and drawing the belly in and up. Then inhale, lifting back up and taking the arms overhead, and exhale, relaxing the arms down to the sides.

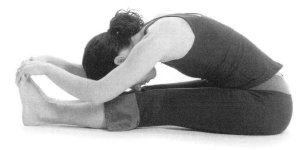

Moderate 50- to 60-Minute Workout

21. Lying Twist (Jathara Parivrtti)

Lie down on the back with the legs long and the arms at the sides. Bend the right knee into the chest, take the left hand to the outside of the right thigh, and extend the right arm out to the side. Exhale and twist to the left, taking the right knee to the floor. Stay for 6 breaths; inhale, easing up, and exhale, deepening the twist and relaxing the right shoulder. Then inhale, bring the right knee back to the chest, switch legs, and repeat the twist to the right side.

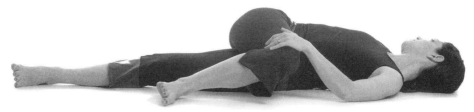

22. Bridge (Setu Bandhasana)

Lie on the back with the knees bent, the feet parallel and hip-width apart, and the arms alongside the body (a). Inhale, lift the arms back overhead, and lift the hips (b). Exhale, take the arms from overhead back alongside the body, and lower the hips. Repeat the breaths and movements four times. Then stay in bridge pose for 6 breaths; inhale, expand through the chest and exhale, letting the belly drop in toward the spine. To release the bridge, exhale, take the arms back from overhead down alongside the body, and lower the hips.

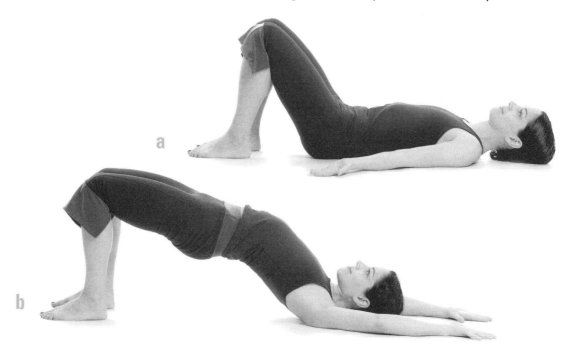

23. Shoulder Stand (Sarvangasana) to Plow (Halasana)

Lie on the back with the knees bent, the feet flat, and the arms alongside the body, palms facing down. If needed, place a blanket under the shoulder and upper back, with the neck off the floor for extra support. Exhale and roll back onto the shoulders, bringing the feet to the floor behind the head *(a)*. With the arms in comfortably close, bend the elbows and place the hands flat on the back. Inhale and lift the legs up to the ceiling. Point through the feet and curl back the toes so that both the front and back of the legs are actively lifting in the shoulder stand *(b)*. Stay lifted for 12 breaths. Then exhale and lower the right knee to the chest, keeping the left leg lifted *(c)*. Inhale, lifting the right leg up, and exhale, lowering the left knee to the chest. Repeat the breathing and movements, alternating two times on each side. Then exhale, lowering both knees to the chest *(d)*, and inhale, lifting the legs back up; repeat four times. Exhale and lower both feet to the floor behind the head and the arms to the floor beside the body. Stay in this plow pose, or halasana, for 6 breaths. Then inhale, roll down to lie on the back, and exhale to rest.

a

b

c

d

24. Corpse (Savasana)

Lie on the back and extend both legs long, with the arms at the sides and the palms facing up. Let go of the breath and of any tension in the body. Let the thoughts come and go freely without allowing them to take you out of the present moment and the sensation of natural breathing for a few minutes.

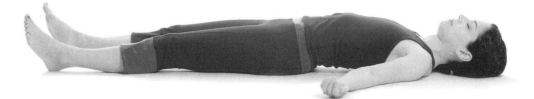

25. Locust (Salabasana)

Roll back over onto the front of the body. With the forehead to the floor, take the arms back along the body and then interlace the fingers together, connecting the palms. Inhale and lift the head, neck, chest, and legs as you reach back through the arms, gazing up. Exhale and relax the head, neck, chest, legs, and forehead back to the floor. Repeat the breathing and movements four times. Then stay lifted in the locust pose for 6 breaths; exhale, letting the belly press into the floor, and inhale, lifting through the chest. Then exhale and relax back down, releasing the hands and placing the palms by the ribs. Inhale, exhale, and come back to child's pose to rest.

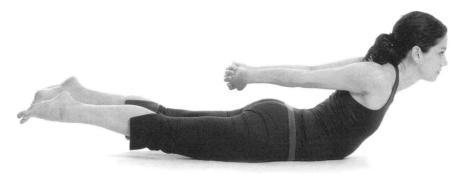

26. Camel (Ustrasana)

Starting in child's pose, take the hands to the back with the palms facing up. Inhale and stand on the knees as you lift the arms up the sides and overhead. Exhale and lower back to child's pose, taking the arms down the sides and the hands to the back. Relax the shoulders. Repeat the breathing and movements four times. Then exhale while you remain standing on the knees and reach the arms behind to hold the heels, curling the toes under if necessary. Holding the heels, inhale and lift through the chest, lengthening the lower back, and exhale, relaxing the head back and staying for 6 breaths. Then inhale, lift the arms overhead, and lift the chest toward the chin. Exhale, come back to child's pose, and rest.

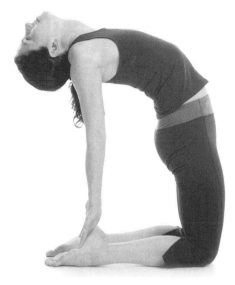

27. Seated Twist (Ardha Matsyendrasana)

Take a seated position with both legs extended forward. Place the right foot to the outside of the left thigh, leaving the left leg long. Place the left arm along the outside of the right thigh and place the right hand, lifted lightly on the fingertips, on the floor behind the body. Soften the gaze to take the focus inward. Inhale, lifting and lengthening the spine, and exhale, engaging the twist to the right, drawing the belly in and up, and turning the head in the same direction. Be mindful not to strain the spine by forcing through the arms and shoulders. Stay in the twist for 6 breaths and then release; repeat the twist to the left.

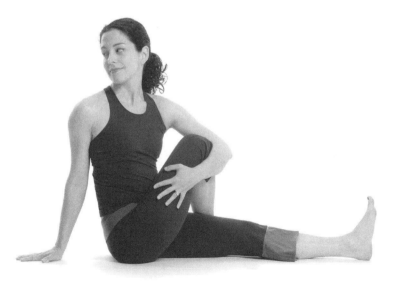

28. Head-to-Knee Forward Bend (Janu Sirsasana)

Sit upright with both legs extended forward. Place the sole of the right foot to the inside of the left thigh, with the right knee out to the side. Pivot the hips and inhale, lifting the arms overhead. Exhale and bend over the extended left leg, placing the hands over the top of the right foot. Relax the head toward the left knee, bending the left knee slightly if necessary. Inhale and lift back up, taking the arms overhead. Then exhale and bend over the left leg again. Repeat the breaths and movements four times. Then stay over the left leg for 6 more breaths; inhale, expanding through the back of the ribs, and exhale, deepening the forward bend. Inhale and lift back up, taking the arms overhead, and exhale, lowering the arms. Switch legs and repeat the asana on the other side.

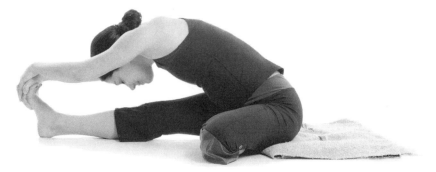

29. Cobbler's Pose (Baddha Konasana)

Sit upright and bring the soles of the feet together in front of the body, close to the groin. Use the hands to open the feet like a book and externally rotate the hips open (a). Holding the feet, inhale and straighten the arms, lengthening the spine. Lower the chin to the chest in jalandhara bandha and stay for 6 breaths, adding a slight pause between the breaths. On the sixth exhalation, round the spine over the legs and extend the arms in front of the body (b) for 6 more breaths. Then walk the arms back and inhale, lifting back up again.

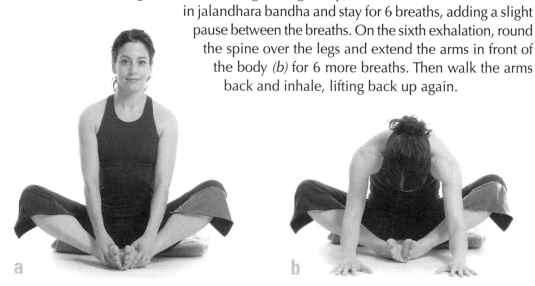

a

b

30. Tabletop

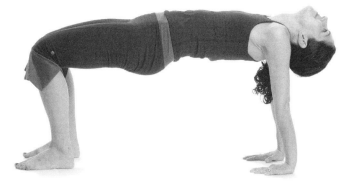

Sitting up with the knees bent, bring the feet flat to the floor and the palms to the floor behind the body, fingers pointed toward the front. Inhale and lift the hips, relaxing the head back and maintaining a solid connection with the floor through both feet. Exhale, lower the hips, and bring the chin toward the chest. Repeat the breathing and movements four times and then stay in tabletop for 6 breaths. Then exhale, lower the hips, and bring the chin to the chest.

31. Alternate Nostril Breathing (Nadi Sodhana Pranayama)

Take a comfortable seated position. Extend the right hand forward with the palm facing up. Bring the index and the middle fingers into the palm. Bring the right hand to the nose, placing the ring finger on the left nostril and the thumb on the right, just below the bridge of the nose. Take one full breath through both nostrils. Then close off the left nostril completely with the ring finger and inhale through the right. Close both nostrils and hold the breath in, lowering the chin toward the chest. Release the ring finger and exhale through the left nostril. Hold the breath out for a few seconds and then inhale through the left nostril. Close both nostrils, hold the breath in for a few seconds, release the right nostril, and exhale to complete one full round of alternate nostril breathing. Repeat nadi sodhana for six full rounds or 12 breaths, finishing with an exhalation through the right nostril. Then relax the right hand down and breathe freely, taking a few minutes to experience the peaceful, clear state of mind.

32. Hand-to-the-Heart Invocation

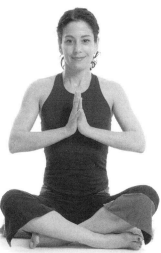

Sit in a cross-legged position with the palms together at the heart and the eyes closed. Inhale and lift the arms up the sides for the palms to meet overhead. Exhale and bring the palms together down to the heart. Repeat the breathing and movements three times to bring a heartfelt sense of openness and receptivity to the start of the day.

Moderate 50- to 60-Minute Workout Guide

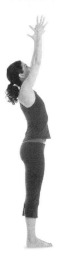

**Breathing Preparations
Mountain**

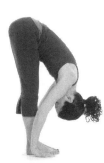

Standing Forward Bend

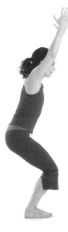

Chair

**Sun Salutation A
See pages 37-38**

**Sun Salutation B
See pages 39-40**

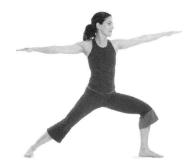

Warrior II

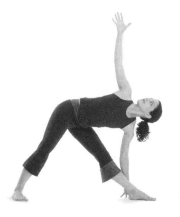

Triangle

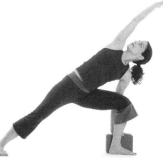

Extended Side Angle

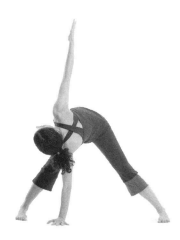

Triangle Twist

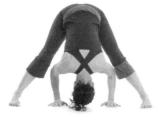

Standing Split Forward Bend

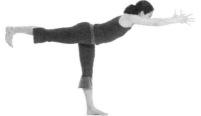

Warrior III

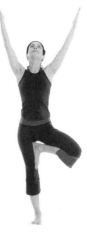

Tree Pose

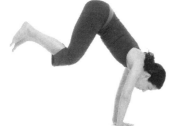

Transition to Cobra

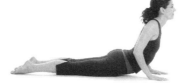

Cobra

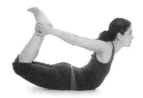

Bow

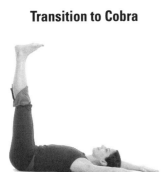

Lying on Back Legs to Sky

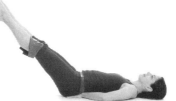

Leg Lifts

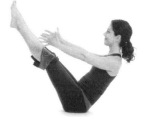

Boat

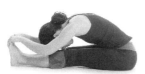

Seated Forward Bend

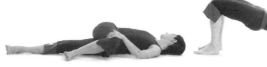

Lying Twist

Bridge

Moderate 50- to 60-Minute Workout Guide

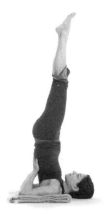

Shoulder Stand to Plow

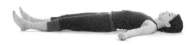

Corpse

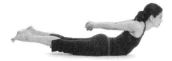

Locust

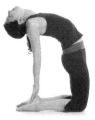

Camel

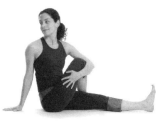

Seated Twist

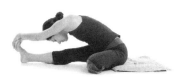

Head-to-Knee Forward Bend

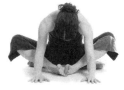

Cobbler's Pose

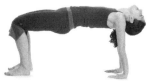

Tabletop

Alternate Nostril Breathing
See page 10

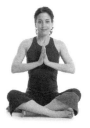

Hand-to-the-Heart Invocation

6

Intense Practice

The intense yoga practices I present here contain the most challenging asanas and vinyasas in the book. These asanas, vinyasas, and breathing techniques require more strength, balance, flexibility, and focus in the bandhas, arm balances, standing postures, deep backbends, and complex inversions. I have purposely excluded asanas that could be overtly hazardous to the joints and body structures, most especially the knees, shoulders, and spine.

Please enjoy these practices sensibly and only when you feel ready and have enough energy. That being said, some of the more intense asanas and vinyasas are fun, invigorating, and liberating; they represent valuable pieces of yoga. For those who are not ready to indulge in this type of yoga asana, don't worry. It can be something to work toward, or not. Be mindful not to overexert or strain beyond your capabilities. As we discussed, the quality of the breath and the conscious combination of breath and body is the real yoga; use them to gauge the quality of practice. The asanas and vinyasas we practice should be enjoyable and playlike. As we explore the boundaries and the edge of our ability to experience more intense variations of yoga asana, the spirit of our yoga should always be lighthearted and open.

Intense 15- to 20-Minute Workout

The 20-minute morning yoga workout is a rush of athletic energy. The variations of poses and sequencing within this practice, as throughout the rest of this chapter, are intended to be challenging. This practice is the essence of high-intensity yoga, when quality of practice takes precedence over quantity.

1. Breathing Preparations

Come to stand at the front of the mat with the feet together and parallel and the arms alongside the body. Soften the gaze and begin to initiate ujjayi breathing through the nose, lengthening the inhalation and deepening the exhalation for 6 breaths.

2. Mountain (Tadasana)

Inhale and lift the arms up the sides for the palms to meet above the head, spreading the fingers wide and gazing up. Exhale and bring the arms down the sides, while lowering the chin toward the chest. Repeat the breath and movements six times.

3. Standing Forward Bend (Uttanasana)

Inhale and lift the arms up the sides for the palms to meet above the head, relaxing the head back and gazing up slightly. Start the exhalation and bend over the legs, bringing the palms to the floor at either side of the feet and the chin toward the chest. Inhale and lift up again as you take the arms up the sides for the palms to meet above the head. Repeat the breathing and movements up and down four times and then stay over in the forward bend for 6 more breaths. Then inhale, lifting back upright and taking the arms up the sides for the palms to meet overhead, and exhale, taking the palms together down the center to meet at the heart.

4. Jumping Sun Salutation

Perform jumping sun salutation as it's described on pages 43–44 in chapter 3.

5. Warrior (Virabhadrasana)

Start standing at the front of the mat with the feet together, the arms at the sides, and the gaze forward. Inhale and lift the arms up the sides for the palms to meet above the head, while gazing up slightly *(a)*. Start the exhalation and bend over the legs, bringing the palms to the floor at either side of the feet *(b)*.

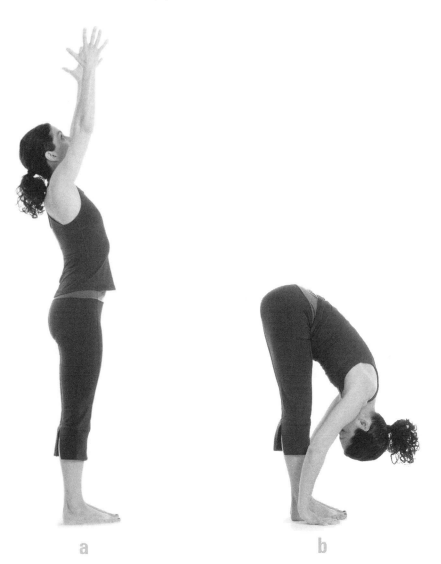

a   b

Intense 15- to 20-Minute Workout

On the pause after the exhalation, step the right foot back, place it down at a 45-degree angle facing forward, and bend the left knee *(c)*. Inhale and take the arms up the sides for the palms to meet above the head, while gazing up *(d)*. Exhale and take the arms back down the sides, bringing the palms to the floor at either side of the front foot, and relax the neck. Inhale and lift back up, taking the arms up the sides for the palms to meet above the head again. Repeat the movements up and down four times, and on the fourth inhalation hold the warrior for 6 breaths. On the sixth exhalation, place the palms down at either side of the left foot. On the pause after the exhalation, step the right foot forward to meet the left at the front of the mat, between the hands, and relax the neck. Inhale and lift up to stand, taking the arms up the sides for the palms to meet above the head. Exhale and take the palms together down to the heart. Repeat the sequence on the other side.

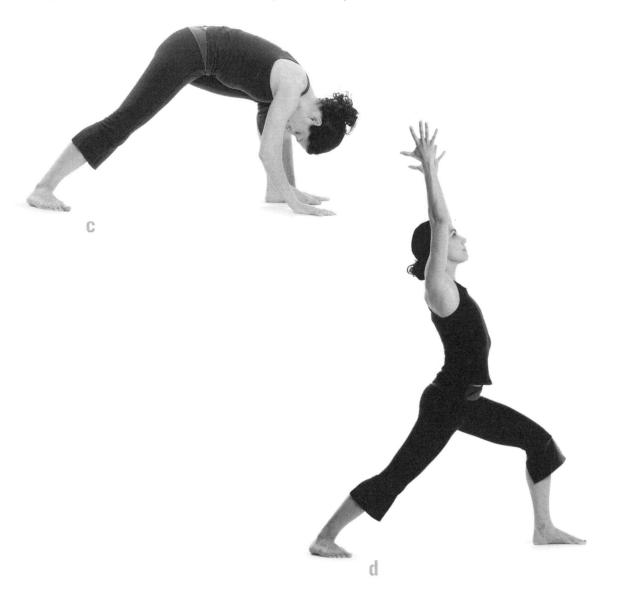

c

d

6. Warrior II (Virabhadrasana II)

Step into a split about four feet long, left leg forward and right leg back, with the left foot at a 45-degree angle toward the front. Open the shoulders to the side and inhale, lifting the arms and extending out through the fingers, with the palms facing down. Exhale and bend the left knee deeply, with a stance long enough that the bent knee does not go beyond the left ankle. Look first over the right hand and ground energy through the right leg as you reach through both arms. Then, maintaining strong energy through both arms and both legs, look forward over the left hand and stay in warrior II for 6 breaths. Inhale and straighten the left leg. Exhale and relax the arms down at the sides. Pivot the feet and repeat warrior II on the other side.

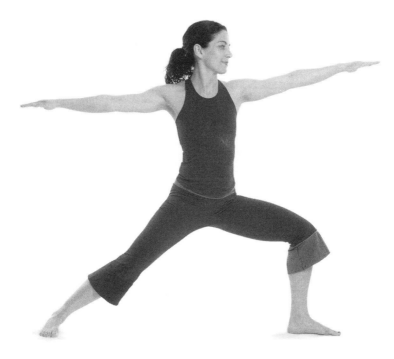

7. Triangle (Trikonasana)

Keep the feet in the same position as the previous warrior pose. Inhale and take the arms out to the sides, reaching through the fingers. With the left leg straight and an unlocked knee, exhale and take the left hand to the outside of the left foot, staying lifted on the fingertips or using a block if needed. Inhale and reach upward through the right arm, with the palm wide, gazing at the right hand. Stay in trikonasana for 6 breaths. Then inhale and lift back upright, reaching through the arms. Exhale, relaxing the arms down, and pivot the feet to repeat triangle on the other side.

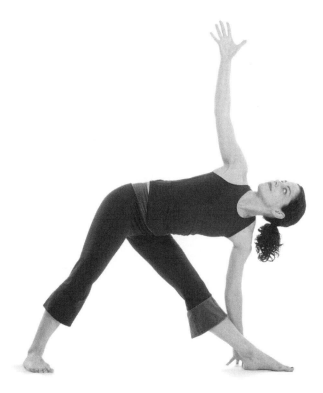

8. Extended Side Angle (Utthita Parsva Konasana) to Half-Moon (Ardha Chandrasana) to One-Sided Standing Forward Bend (Parsva Uttanasana)

In a split stance with the right foot forward and the left leg back, inhale and reach the arms out to the sides. Exhale, bend the left knee, and place the left hand at the inside of the left shin, or on a block placed on the outside of the left foot, and the right hand on the right hip. Rotate the left thigh open and the left hip back. Grounding through the right leg, reach the right arm forward into utthita parsva konasana, extended side angle *(a)*, gazing either directly up into the armpit or straight to the side, for 6 breaths. On the sixth exhalation take the right hand to the right hip and look down at the left foot. To come into half-moon pose, place the hand on a block slightly further in front of the outside of the left foot and come up on the fingertips. Inhale, lifting the right leg up with the right foot parallel to the floor, and exhale, straightening the left leg. Inhale, open the chest to the side, and lift the right arm up, spreading the palm and fingers wide and looking either to the side or the right hand *(b)*. Stay in this half-moon pose for 6 breaths.

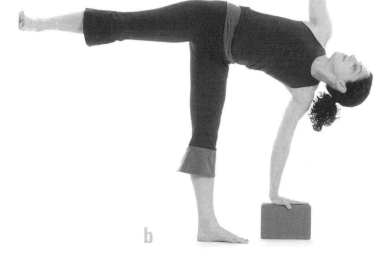

On the sixth exhalation lower the right leg, placing the right foot at a 45-degree angle facing forward and the hands to either side of the left foot. Inhale, lengthen the spine, and rotate the hips and shoulders forward. Exhale, bend over the left leg, bringing the head toward the left knee, and stay in parsva uttanasana *(c)* for 6 breaths. Then with a straight left leg, inhale and lift the arms overhead *(d)*. Exhale and lower the arms to the sides. Switch legs and repeat this vinyasa on the other side.

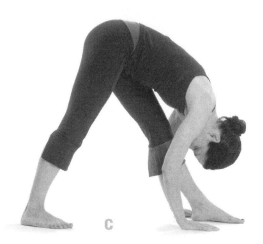

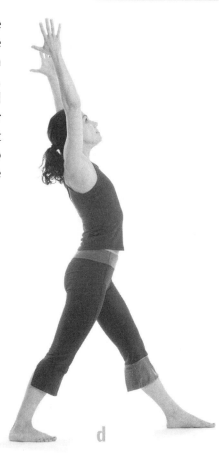

9. Chair (Utkatasana) and Transition to Kneeling

Step to the front of the mat with the feet hip-width apart and parallel and the arms at the sides. Gazing forward, inhale and lift the arms up the sides and above the head, keeping the palms separate and parallel. Exhale, bend the knees, lower the hips, and place the palms to the floor in front of the body *(a)*. Be sure to round the spine and relax the neck. Keep the heels on the floor if possible; lift them if you need to or place a blanket under the heels at the beginning of the sequence.

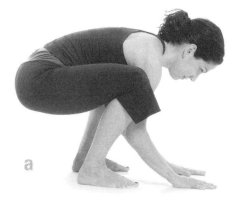

b

c

d

e

Inhale and lift the arms up the front of the body and above the head as you lift the chest and straighten the legs. Repeat the breaths and movements up and down six times. On the pause after the sixth exhalation, place the hands to either side of the feet and gently hop back *(b)* to a low push-up in chataranga dandasana, or stick pose, keeping the toes curled under. Here the chest and thighs should be in line and lifted off the floor, with the elbows in close to the body, and the shoulders back *(c)*. Inhale and pivot the hips forward to upward-facing dog *(d)*. Exhale and pivot back to downward-facing dog *(e)* for 5 breaths. Then inhale, lower the knees to the floor, lift the chest, and look up slightly.

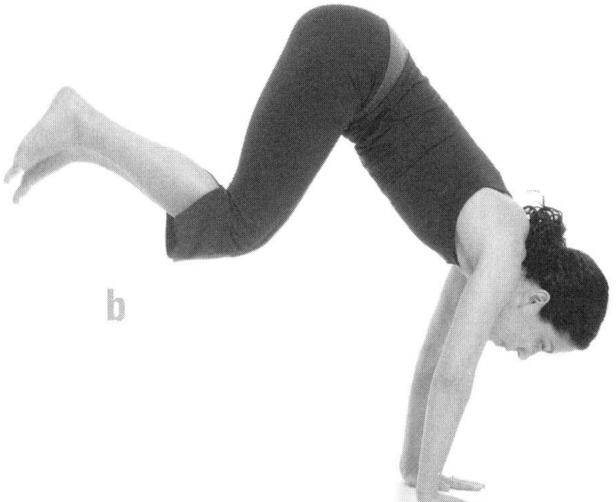

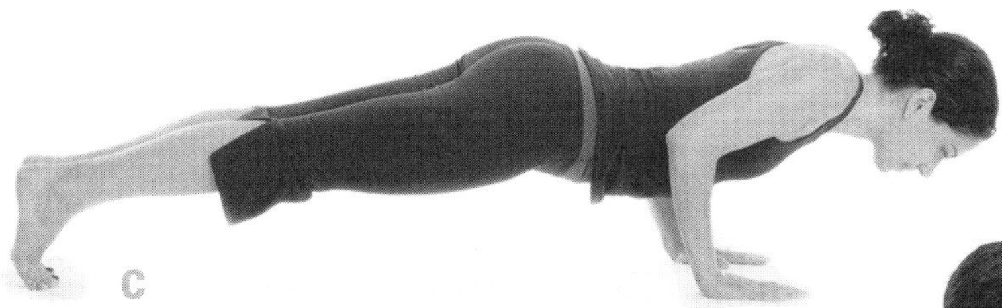

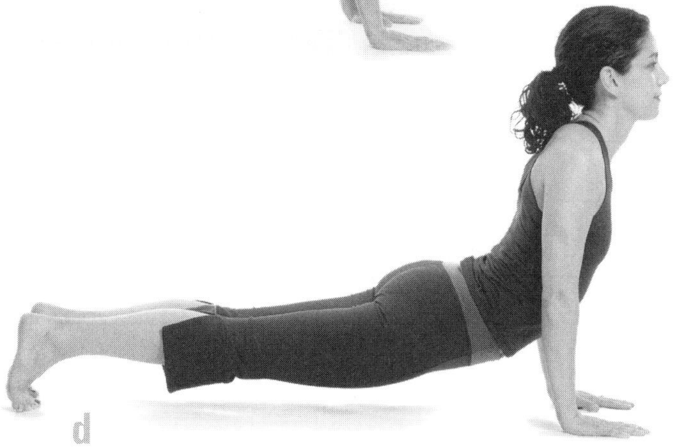

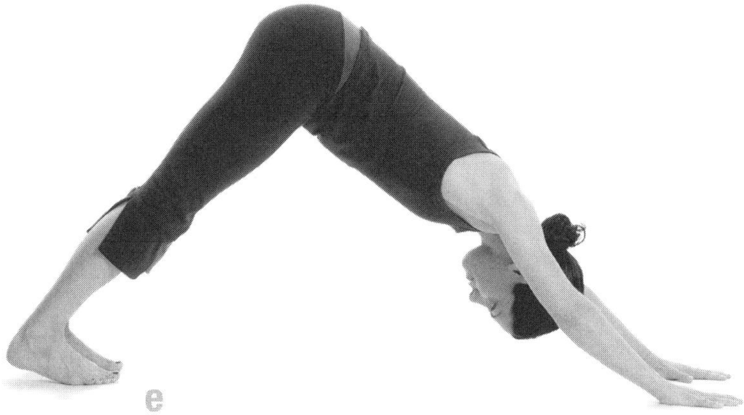

10. Pigeon (Eka Pada Kapotasana) to Downward-Facing Dog (Adho Mukha Svanasana)

Start on the hands and knees. Slide the left leg forward, place the shin to the floor at an angle, keeping the front knee and hip in one line, and extend back through the right leg. If you need to, use a blanket under the lifted left hip. Place the hands at either side of the

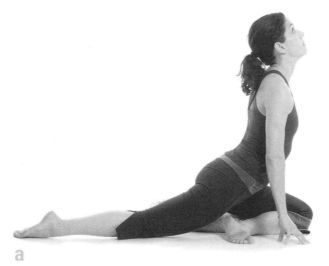

left knee and inhale, lifting the chest to a back arch, straightening the arms, and looking up slightly (a). Exhale, bend the elbows, and lower the forehead to the floor. Repeat the breaths and movements three times. Then exhale, extending the arms out in front of the body and staying in pigeon pose over the leg (b) for 6 breaths. Walk the hands back to either side of the left knee. Inhale, straighten the arms, and lift the chest. Then bend the right leg, hold the inside of the right foot with the right hand, lift up onto the fingertips of the left hand, and open the shoulders to the right (c) for 6 more breaths.

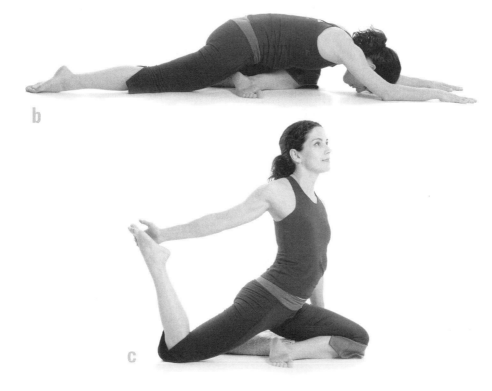

Release the ankle and bring the right hand back to the floor, curl the toes of the right foot under, and exhale back to downward-facing dog *(d)* for 5 breaths. Then lower both knees to the floor, lift the chest, and repeat the vinyasa on the other side.

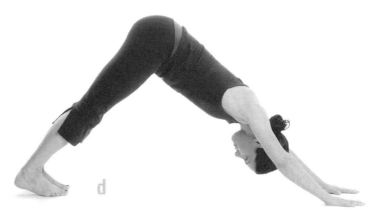

11. Child's Pose (Balasana) to Standing on Knees to Camel (Ustrasana)

Exhale and come back to child's pose *(a)*. Inhale and stand on the knees, reaching the arms up the front of the body to overhead and gazing up slightly. Exhale and come back to child's pose, lowering the arms down the front of the body. Repeat the breathing and movements four times. On the fourth exhalation remain standing on the knees and take the arms back to hold the heels in ustrasana, camel *(b)*. Inhale and lift through the chest while lengthening the lower back. Exhale, relax the head back fully, and stay for 6 breaths. Then inhale, lifting back up as you take the arms above the head. Exhale, come back to child's pose, and rest.

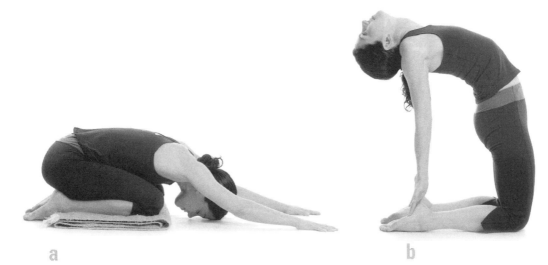

12. Child's Pose (Balasana) to Cat

Start in child's pose *(a)* with the arms extending in front of the body. Inhale and come up to the hands and knees, lifting the chest into a slight back arch, looking up slightly *(b)*. Exhale and come back to child's pose. Repeat the breathing and movements six times.

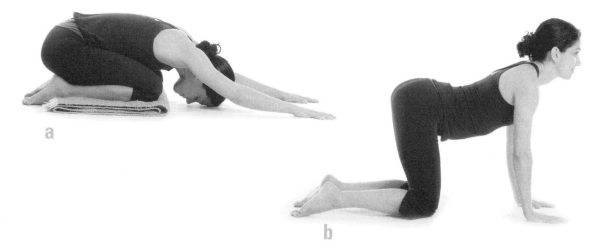

13. Boat (Navasana)

Come up to sit, bringing the legs around in front of the body with knees bent and feet flat on the floor. Inhale, extending the arms forward of the body, and exhale, lifting the feet off the floor. Inhale, straighten the legs, and point through the feet. Stay in navasana, balancing on the buttocks with the upper back rounded slightly, for 6 breaths. Then inhale, lower the legs to the floor in front of the body, and place the hands alongside the hips.

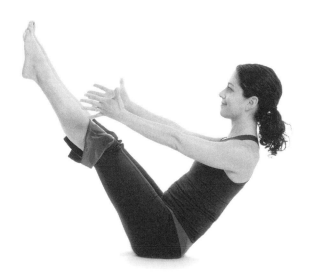

14. Seated Forward Bend (Pascimatanasana)

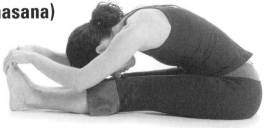

Remain seated upright with the legs extended in front of the body and the hands at the hips. Inhale, lifting the arms overhead, and exhale, bending over the legs, placing the hands over the feet, and relaxing the neck. Inhale and lift back up, taking the arms overhead and keeping the chin lowered to the chest. Exhale, bending over the legs again. Repeat the breathing and movements up and down four times. Then stay over the legs in pascimatanasana for 6 more breaths; inhale, expanding through the ribs and back of the body, and exhale, deepening into the forward bend and drawing the belly in toward the spine. Then inhale and lift back up, taking the arms overhead, and exhale, relaxing the arms down to the sides.

15. Seated Twist (Ardha Matsyendrasana)

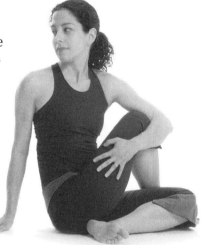

Start seated with both legs extended in front of the body. Place the right foot to the outside of the left thigh. Then bend the right leg toward the body and place the left arm around the right thigh and the right hand to the floor behind the body. Remain grounded through both hips and soften the gaze. Inhale, lengthening the spine, and exhale, twisting toward the right and looking over the right shoulder. Stay in the twist for 6 breaths; inhale, lengthening the spine, and exhale, deepening the twist and drawing the belly in and up. Then inhale, release forward, and repeat the twist to the left side.

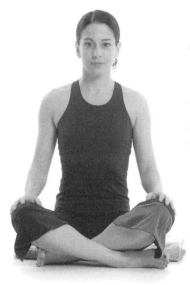

16. Easy Cross-Legged Seated Pose (Sukhasana)

Take a seated cross-legged position with the inside sole of the foot close to the groin and the hands on the knees, palms facing up. Bring the index finger to touch the thumb. Close the eyes and take a few moments to breath consciously and absorb the benefits of the practice.

Intense 15- to 20-Minute Workout Guide

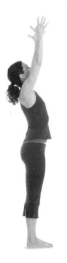

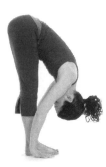

**Breathing Preparations
Mountain**

Standing Forward Bend

**Jumping Sun Salutation
See page 44**

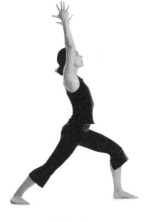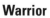

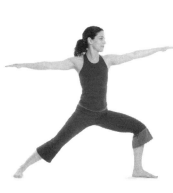

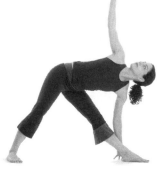

Warrior

Warrior II

Triangle

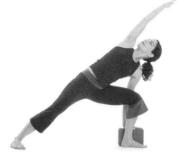

Extended Side Angle Vinyasa
Switch legs and
repeat on other side

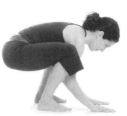

Chair and
Transition to Kneeling

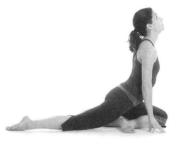

Pigeon to
Downward-Facing Dog

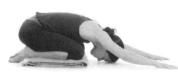

Child's Pose Vinyasa

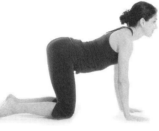

Child's Pose to Cat

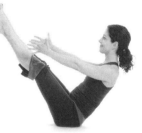

Boat

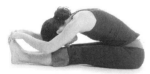

Seated Forward Bend

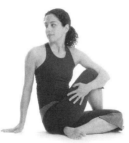

Seated Twist

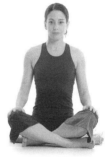

Easy Cross-Legged
Seated Pose

Intense 30- to 40-Minute Workout

The 40-minute intense morning yoga workout builds on the shorter previous practice. It is similar in pacing but packed with even more challenging pose variations within an invigorating sequence.

1. Breathing Preparations

Stand at the front of the mat with the feet together and the arms alongside the body. Soften the gaze and begin to initiate ujjayi breathing through the nose, lengthening the inhalation and deepening the exhalation for 6 breaths.

2. Mountain (Tadasana)

Inhale and lift the arms up the sides for the palms to meet above the head, spreading the fingers wide and gazing up. Exhale and bring the arms down the sides while lowering the chin toward the chest. Repeat the breathing and movements six times.

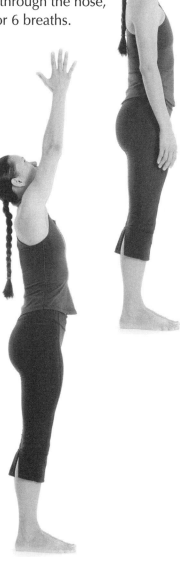

3. Standing Forward Bend (Uttanasana)

Inhale and lift the arms up the sides for the palms to meet above the head, relaxing the head back and gazing up slightly. Start the exhalation and bend over the legs, bringing the palms to the floor at either side of the feet and the chin toward the chest. Inhale and lift up as you take the arms up the sides for the palms to meet above the head again. Repeat the breathing and movements up and down four times and then stay over in the forward bend for 6 more breaths. Then inhale and lift back upright, taking the arms up the sides for the palms to meet above head. Exhale and take the palms together down the center to meet at the heart.

4. Sun Salutation With Lunge

Perform sun salutation with lunge as it's described on pages 40–42 in chapter 3.

5. Jumping Sun Salutation

Perform jumping sun salutation as it's described on pages 43–44 in chapter 3.

6. Warrior I (Virabhadrasana I) to Warrior II (Virabhadrasana II) to Triangle (Trikonasana) to Extended Side Angle (Utthita Parsva Konasana) to Half-Moon Pose (Ardha Chandrasana) to One-Sided Standing Forward Bend (Parsva Uttanasana) to Warrior III (Virabhadrasana III) to Standing

Start at the front of the mat with the feet parallel and at hip-width distance, the arms at the sides, and the gaze forward. Inhale and take the arms up the sides for the palms to meet above the head. Exhale and bend over the legs, placing the palms to the floor at either side of the feet. Holding the breath out, step the right leg back about four feet and place the foot down at a 45-degree angle, facing forward *(a)*. Inhale, bend the left knee, and take the arms up the sides for the palms to meet above the head in warrior I *(b)*. Hold for 6 breaths.

Intense 30- to 40-Minute Workout

Then exhale and come into warrior II, opening the arms and shoulders to the right, reaching through the fingers with the palms facing down, and gazing forward *(c)* for 6 breaths. To come into triangle, inhale and straighten the left leg. Then exhale and extend forward, placing the left hand on the left shin or to the outside of the left foot, using a block if needed. Inhale, lifting through the right arm and looking at the right hand, and hold the triangle *(d)* for 6 breaths. To come into utthita parsva konasana, exhale and bend the left knee, grounding through both feet. Then inhale and reach the right arm forward for 6 more breaths, gazing either forward or up *(e)*.

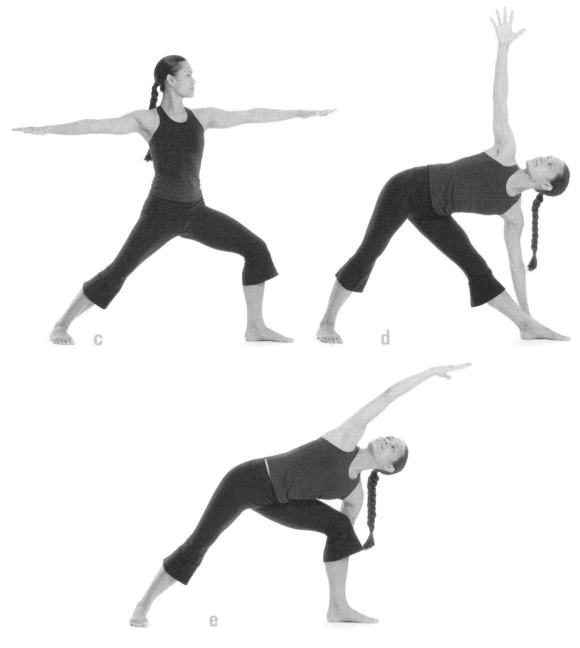

To come into half-moon, or ardha chandrasana, place the right hand on the right hip and inhale, lifting the right leg. Exhale, straightening the left leg, and inhale, rotating the torso open to the side, lifting the right arm directly up, and looking at the right hand *(f)*. Stay in half-moon for 6 breaths. Then exhale, lower the right leg back down, position the right foot at a 45-degree angle forward, and place the hands on either side of the left foot. Inhale, lengthening the spine and rotating the hips and shoulders forward. Then exhale and straighten the left leg into parsva uttanasana *(g)*, staying for 6 breaths.

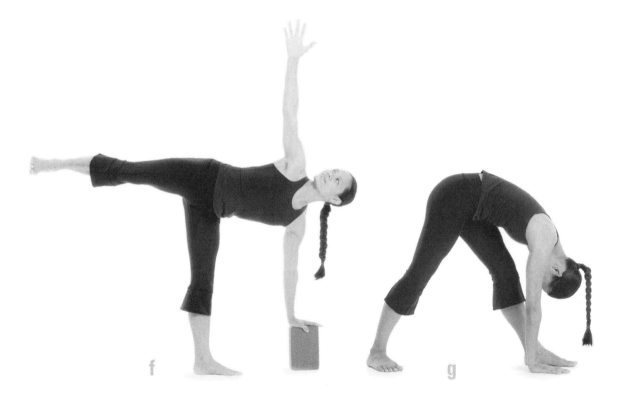

Intense 30- to 40-Minute Workout

To come into warrior III, bring both hands to the hips, and bend the left leg slightly. Inhale and lift the right leg, keeping the right leg and the chest parallel and the keeping the right foot and the hips perpendicular to the floor. Exhale, straightening the left leg, and inhale, extending the arms in front of the body *(h)*. Stay in warrior III for 6 breaths. Then inhale and lift up to standing with the arms over head as the right foot comes down to meet the left. Exhale and bring the palms together to the heart. Repeat the full vinyasa on the other side.

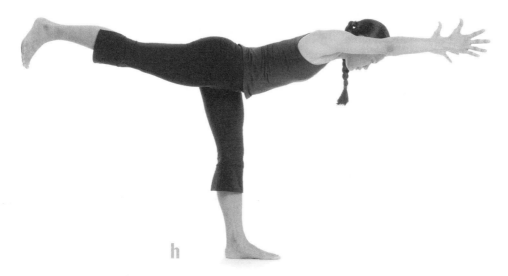

h

7. Triangle Twist (Parivrtti Trikonasana)

Stand in a split on the mat with the feet parallel and the arms at the sides. Inhale and reach the arms out to the sides *(a)*. Exhale and twist to the right, placing the left hand on the outside of the right foot, extending the right arm up, and gazing at the right hand *(b)*. Inhale and lift back to center, reaching through both arms. Exhale and twist toward the left, placing the right hand to the outside of the left foot and lifting the left arm up, gazing at the left hand. Inhale, reaching through the arms, and lift back to center. Repeat the twist four times to each side and then stay for 6 breaths on each side. After staying on both sides inhale, reaching through the arms and lifting to center, and exhale, lowering the arms and relaxing.

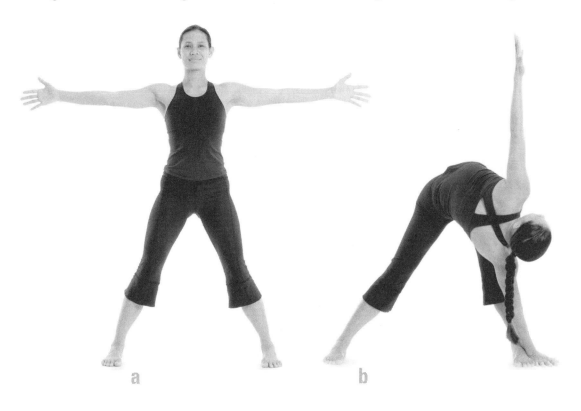

a   b

8. Prayer at Heart in Squat (Namaskarasana) to Crow (Bakasana)

Step to the front of the mat, gazing forward, with the feet hip-width apart and parallel and the arms at the sides. Inhale and take the arms overhead, keeping the palms separate and parallel. Exhale and bend the knees, lowering the hips, rounding the spine, and bringing the palms to the floor in front of the body (a). Open the hips and squeeze the outside of the upper arms with the inside of the thighs. Lift the chest, place the hands together at the heart (b), and stay in the namaskarasana squat for 6 breaths. Then exhale, place the hands back down to the floor in front of the body, and continue to press the inside of the thighs against the outside of the upper arms (a). Inhale and shift forward, coming up onto the toes while gazing forward. Take one full breath and then, on the pause after the exhalation, draw the belly in and up into mula bandha, lifting the feet off the floor to balance on the hands in bakasana, crow pose (c). Stay for 6 breaths, maintaining the deep use of the abdominal musculature.

a

b

c

9. Jump Back to Stick (Chataranga Dandasana) to Upward-Facing Dog (Urdva Mukha Svanasana) to Downward-Facing Dog (Adho Mukha Svanasana) to Jump Through to Sit

From crow, on the pause after the last exhalation, lightly jump back to a low push-up in chataranga dandasana, or stick pose, keeping the toes curled under *(a)*. Here the body should be lifted a few inches off the floor, with the elbows in close to the body and the shoulders back. Inhale and pivot the hips forward to upward-facing dog *(b)*. Then exhale to downward-facing dog for 4 breaths *(c)*. On the pause after the last exhalation, lift onto the fingertips and hop the legs forward through the arms *(d)*, coming to sit with the legs extended in front of the body *(e)*.

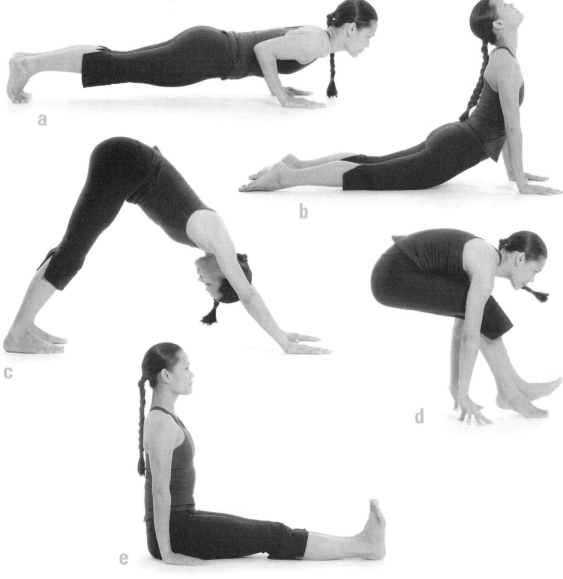

10. Boat (Navasana)

Sitting upright, bend the knees with the feet flat on the floor. Inhale, reaching the arms out in front of the body, and exhale, lifting the feet off the floor. Inhale, straightening the legs and pointing through the feet, and stay in navasana for 6 breaths. Then inhale, lower the legs to the floor in front of the body, and place the hands alongside the hips.

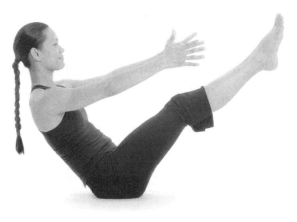

11. Seated Forward Bend (Pascimatanasana)

Sit upright with the legs extended in front of the body and the hands placed along the hips. Inhale, lifting the arms overhead (a), and exhale, bending over the legs, placing the hands over the feet , and relaxing the neck (b). Inhale and lift back up, taking the arms overhead, and exhale, bending over the legs again. Repeat the breathing and movements four times. Then stay over the legs in pascimatanasana for 6 more breaths; inhale, expanding through the ribs and the back of the body, and exhale, deepening into the forward bend and drawing the belly in toward the spine. Inhale and lift back upright, taking the arms overhead, and exhale, relaxing the arms down the sides.

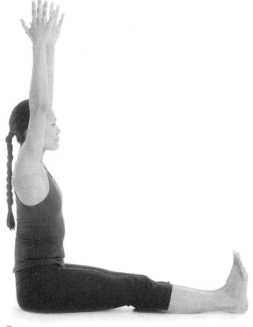

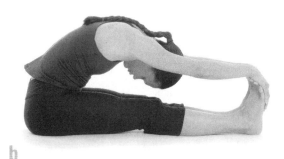

a

b

12. Seated Twist (Ardha Matsyendrasana)

Start seated, with both legs extended in front of the body. Place the right foot to the outside of the left thigh, bending the right leg toward the body, placing the left arm around the right thigh, and putting the right hand on the floor behind the body. Remain grounded through both hips and soften the gaze. Inhale, lengthening the spine, and exhale, twisting to the right and looking over the right shoulder. Stay in the twist for 6 breaths; inhale, lengthening the spine, and exhale, deepening the twist and drawing the belly in and up. Then inhale, release forward, and repeat the twist to the left.

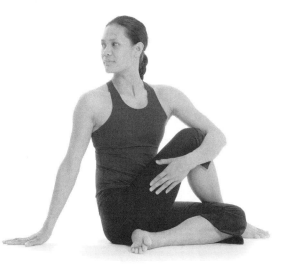

13. Cobbler's Pose (Baddha Konasana)

Sit upright and bring the soles of the feet together in front of the body, close to the groin. Use the hands to open the feet like a book and externally rotate the hips open. Holding the feet, inhale and straighten the arms, lengthening the spine and lowering the chin to the chest in jalandhara bandha *(a)*. Stay for 6 breaths, adding a slight pause between the breaths. On the sixth exhalation, round the spine over the legs and extend the arms in front of the body *(b)* for 6 more breaths. Then walk the arms back and inhale, lifting back upright.

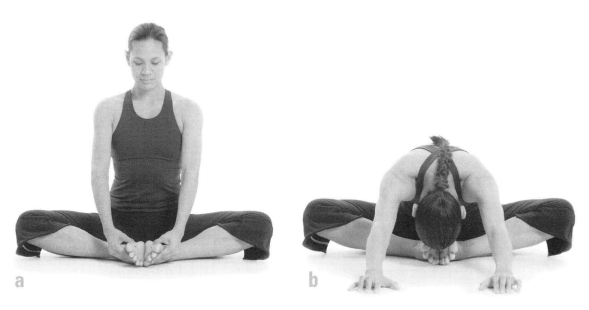

a

b

14. Bridge (Setu Bandhasana)

Lie on the back with the knees bent, the feet parallel and hip-width apart, and the arms alongside the body *(a)*. Inhale, lift the arms back overhead, and lift the hips *(b)*. Exhale, take the arms from overhead back alongside the body, and lower the hips. Repeat the breath and movements four times. Then stay in bridge for 6 breaths; inhale, opening through the heart and exhale, letting the belly drop in toward the spine. Exhale, take the arms back down from overhead to alongside the body, and lower the hips.

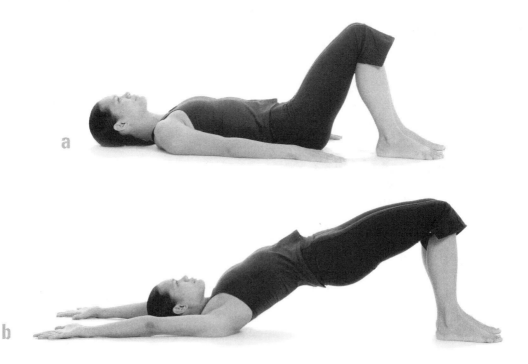

15. Wheel (Urdva Danurasana)

Lie on the back with the knees bent and the feet hip-width apart and parallel. Place the palms flat by the ears, with the fingers toward the body *(a)*. Exhale, press through the feet, and extend through the arms, lifting into urdva danurasana and relaxing the head back completely *(b)*. Stay in wheel for 8 breaths, distributing the weight through the upper body as well as grounding through the front of the feet to prevent lower-back and shoulder strain. On the last exhalation, tuck in the chin and then bend and lower back down to rest.

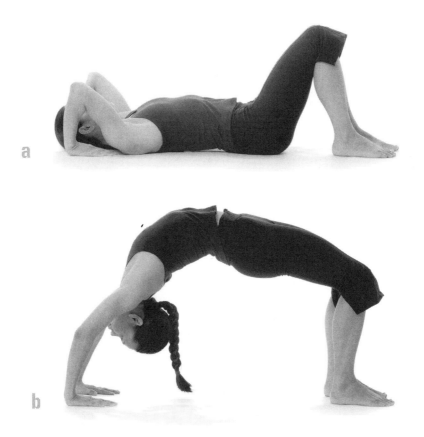

Intense 30- to 40-Minute Workout

16. Lying on Back Legs to Sky (Urdva Prasarita Padasana)

Lie on the back and hug in the knees, with one hand on each knee *(a)*. Inhale, take the arms back overhead, and extend the legs directly up while flexing the feet *(b)*. Exhale and hug in the knees again. Repeat the breathing and movements four times, and then stay for 6 breaths with the legs lifted and the arms back. Exhale and hug in the knees to relax.

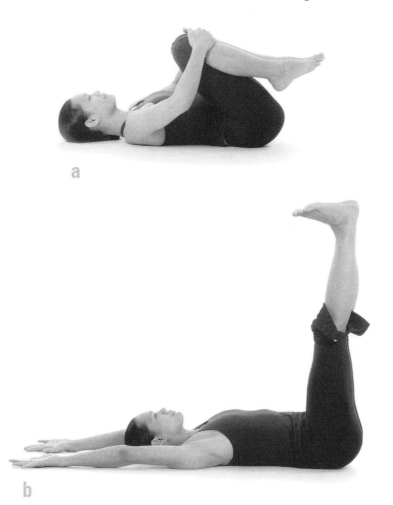

a

b

17. Headstand (Sirsasana)

Come onto the hands and knees. Measure that the elbows are at a forearm's length apart, and interlace the fingers to form a cradle for the head. Place the back of the top of the head to the floor between the interlaced fingers. Curl the toes under, lift the hips, and walk the feet forward toward the elbows until the hips are lifted above the torso *(a)*. Balancing on the forearms and hands, with very little pressure on the head, bend the knees to the chest *(b)* and inhale, lifting the legs to stay in the headstand *(c)* for 12 breaths. Exhale and lower the legs straight to the floor. Bend the knees and release the head from the hands, then come back to child's pose and rest. Note that you can do this pose by a wall for added support at first.

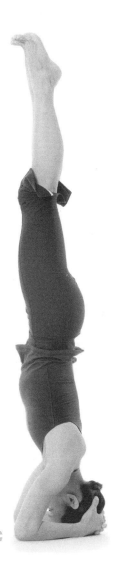
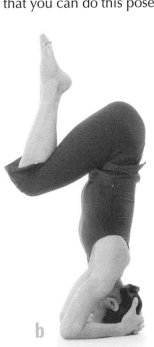
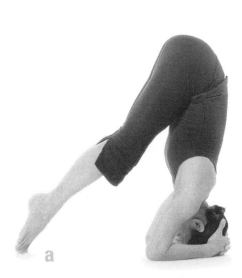

a

b

c

Intense 30- to 40-Minute Workout

18. Shoulder Stand (Sarvangasana) to Plow (Halasana)

Come from child's pose to lie on the back with the knees bent, the feet flat, and the arms alongside the body, palms facing down. For extra support place a blanket under the shoulder and upper back, with the neck off the floor. Exhale and roll back onto the shoulders, bringing the feet to the floor behind the head *(a)*. With the arms in comfortably close, bend the elbows and place the hands flat on the back. Inhale and lift the legs up to the ceiling. Point through the feet and curl back the toes so that both the front and back of the legs are actively lifting in the shoulder stand *(b)*. Stay lifted for 12 breaths. Then exhale and lower the right knee to the chest, keeping the left leg lifted *(c)*. Inhale, lifting the right leg up, and exhale, lowering the left knee to the chest. Repeat the breathing and movements, alternating two times on each side. Then exhale, lowering both knees to the chest *(d)*, and inhale, lifting the legs back up; repeat four times. Exhale and lower both feet to the floor behind the head and the arms to the floor beside the body. Stay in halasana, or plow, for 6 breaths. Then inhale, roll down to lie on your back, and exhale to rest.

a

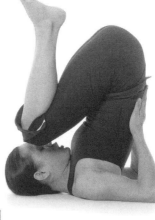

b

c

d

19. Corpse Pose (Savasana)

Lie on the back and extend both legs long, with the arms at the sides and the palms facing up. Let go of the breath and any tension in the body. Let the thoughts come and go freely without allowing them to take you out of the present moment and the sensation of natural breathing for a few minutes.

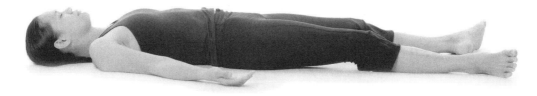

20. Cobra (Bhujangasana)

Roll over onto the front of the body to lie face down. Bring the palms flat next to the ribs, with the elbows lifted. Inhale, pressing into the hands, lifting the head, neck, and chest, and looking up slightly. Exhale and relax the head, neck, and chest back to the floor. Repeat the breaths and movements four times. Then stay lifted in cobra for 6 breaths; exhale, letting the belly press into the floor, and inhale, lifting up slightly and expanding through the chest. On the sixth exhalation relax the head, neck, and chest back to the floor. Inhale here and then exhale back to child's pose.

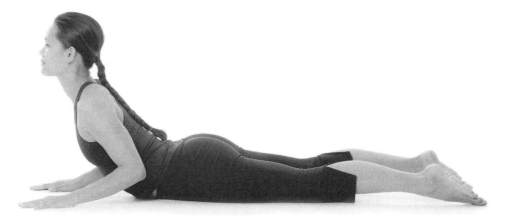

21. Child's Pose (Balasana) to Cat

Start in child's pose *(a)* with the arms extending in front of the body. Inhale and come up to the hands and knees, lifting the chest into a back arch, looking up slightly *(b)*. Exhale and come back to child's pose. Repeat the breathing and movement six times.

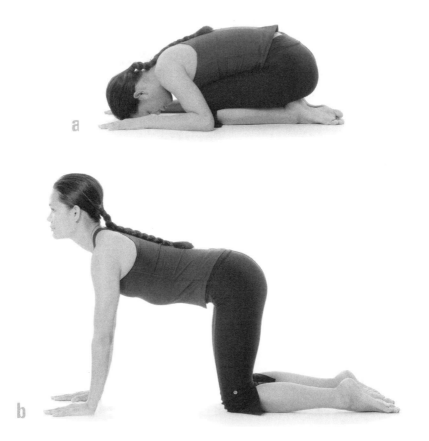

22. Seated Ocean Breathing (Ujjayi Pranayama) With Bandha

Take a comfortable seated position with the arms extended, the palms on the knees facing up, and the chest lifted toward the chin. Close the eyes and form a mudra, or energetic hand gesture, by touching the index finger and the thumb and extending the other fingers long with both hands. Inhale for 8 seconds using ocean breathing and then lower the chin toward the chest to hold the breath in for 5 seconds. Keep a long spine and exhale for 8 seconds, drawing the belly in and up. Lower the chin again, lift the chest, and hold the breath out for 5 seconds. Repeat this breath ratio for 4 breaths and then lengthen the next inhalation to 12 seconds. Hold the breath in for 8 seconds. Deepen the exhalation to 12 seconds. Now, on the pause after the exhalation, lower the chin, lift the chest, and scoop the belly under the ribs to initiate udayana bandha and experience mula and jalandhara bandha together for 8 seconds. Ease up and release the diaphragm, abdomen, and throat slightly prior to the next inhalation. Repeat this breathing technique and ratio for 10 more breaths and then go back to the initial ratio of 8-second inhalation, 5-second pause, 8-second exhalation, 5-second pause for another 4 breaths. To finish the pranayama, breathe freely for a few moments and observe the breath coming and going with ease. Take a moment to fully experience your state of being prior to starting the rest of your day.

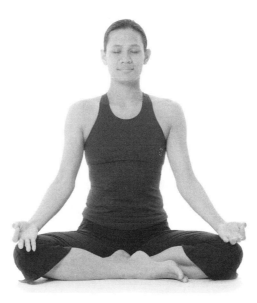

Intense 30- to 40-Minute Workout Guide

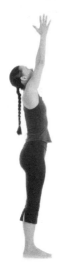

**Breathing Preparations
Mountain**

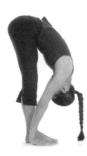

Standing Forward Bend

**Sun Salutation With Lunge
See pages 40-42**

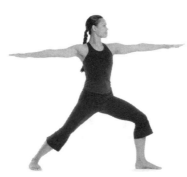

**Jumping Sun Salutation
See page 44**

**Warrior I Vinyasa
Repeat on the other side.**

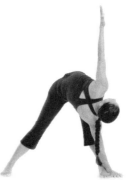

Triangle Twist

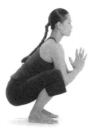

**Prayer at Heart
in Squat to Crow**

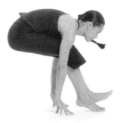

Jump Back to Stick Vinyasa

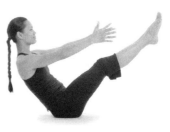

Boat

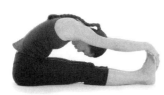

Seated Forward Bend

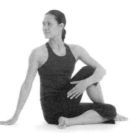

Seated Twist

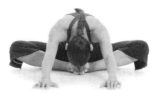

Cobbler's Pose

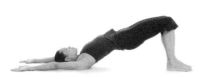

Bridge

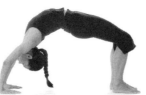

Wheel

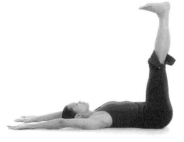

Lying on Back Legs to Sky

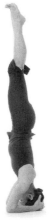

Headstand

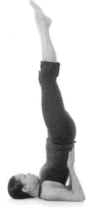

Shoulder Stand to Plow

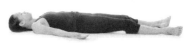

Corpse Pose

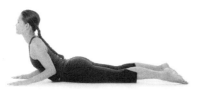

Cobra

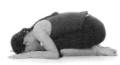

Child's Pose to Cat

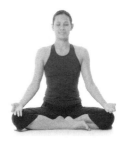

**Seated Ocean Breathing
With Bandha**

Intense 50- to 60-Minute Workout

The 60-minute intense morning yoga workout is the apex of physical challenge—a culmination of all of the poses and sequences that have come before it. Not appropriate for everyone all of the time, the 60-minute practice requires deep concentration and a willingness to play to the edge of our limits.

1. Breathing Preparations

Stand at the front of the mat with the feet together and the arms alongside the body. Soften the gaze and begin to initiate ujjayi breathing through the nose, lengthening the inhalation and deepening the exhalation for 6 breaths.

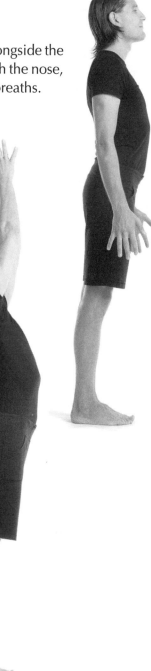

2. Mountain (Tadasana)

Inhale and lift the arms up the sides for the palms to meet above the head, spreading the fingers wide and gazing up. Exhale and bring the arms down the sides while lowering the chin toward the chest. Repeat the breathing and movements six times.

3. Standing Forward Bend (Uttanasana)

Inhale and lift the arms up the sides for the palms to meet above the head, relaxing the head back and gazing up slightly. Start the exhalation and bend over the legs, bringing the palms to the floor at either side of the feet and lowering the chin toward the chest. Inhale and lift up as you take the arms up the sides for the palms to meet above the head again. Repeat the breathing and movements up and down four times and then stay over in the forward bend for 6 more breaths. Inhale and lift back upright, taking the arms up the sides for the palms to meet overhead. Exhale and take the palms together down the center to meet at the heart.

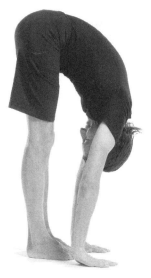

4. Chair (Utkatasana)

Remain standing at the front of the mat, gazing forward, with the feet together and parallel and the arms at the sides. Inhale and lift the arms up the sides to overhead, keeping the palms separate and parallel and lowering the chin toward the chest. Exhale and bend the knees, lowering the hips, rounding the spine, and taking the hands to the floor in front of the body *(a)*. The heels stay on the floor or on a blanket. Keeping the knees bent, inhale and lift the arms and torso again *(b)*. Exhale, round the spine, and bring the hands to the floor. Then inhale and lift back up to stand, taking the arms overhead. Exhale and lower the arms down the sides. Repeat the breaths and the movements four times and then stay in utkatasana with the knees bent, the chest lifted, and the arms above the head for 6 breaths. Inhale and straighten the legs, keeping the arms above the head. Then exhale, lower the arms down to the sides, and relax.

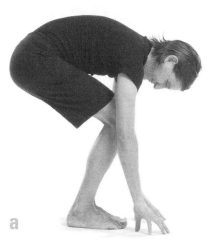

a

b

5. Sun Salutation with Lunge

Perform sun salutation with lunge as it's described on pages 40–42 in chapter 3.

6. Warrior I (Virabhadrasana I) to Warrior II (Virabhadrasana II) to Triangle (Trikonasana) to Extended Side Angle (Utthita Parsva Konasana) to One-Sided Standing Forward Bend (Parsva Uttanasana) to Warrior III (Virabhadrasana III)

Stand at the front of the mat with the feet hip-width apart, the arms at the sides, and the gaze forward. Inhale and lift the arms up the sides for the palms to meet above the head, while you look up slightly (a). Exhale and bend over the legs, placing the hands at either side of the feet (b). On the pause after the exhalation, step the right foot back to a long split and place it down at a 45-degree angle, facing forward (c).

a   b   c

Inhale, lifting the arms up the sides to meet above the head in warrior I *(d)*. Exhale and bend over the left leg, placing the hands beside the left foot again and relaxing the neck completely. Inhale, lift back up to warrior I, and repeat the breathing and movements four times. Then stay lifted in warrior I for 6 more breaths. On the sixth exhalation, open the arms and shoulders to the right and come into warrior II *(e)*, gazing forward and reaching through the arms and fingers with the palms facing down, for 6 breaths.

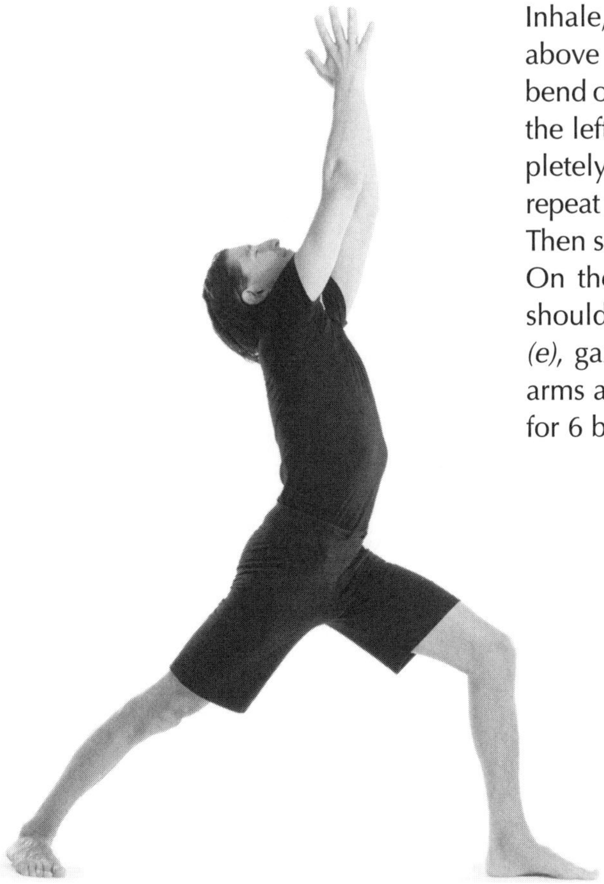

d

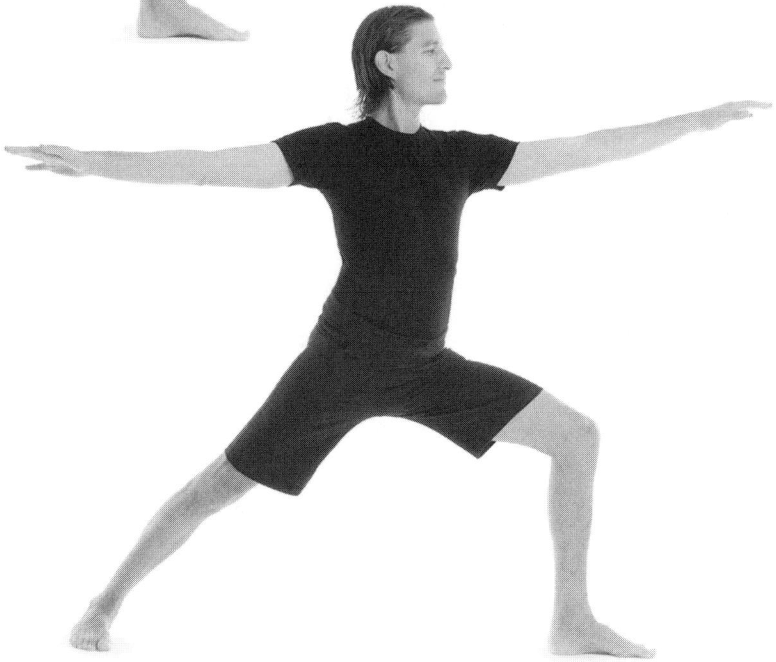

e

Then inhale and straighten the left leg. Exhale and extend over the left leg into triangle, placing the left hand on the left shin or on the outside of the left foot, lifting through the right arm, and looking up *(f)*. Hold for 6 breaths. Exhale and bend the left knee. Inhale and reach the right arm forward over the right ear into extended side angle, utthita parsva konasana *(g)*, for 6 more breaths, gazing directly up and grounding through both feet, with the left hand on the outside of the left foot or on a block.

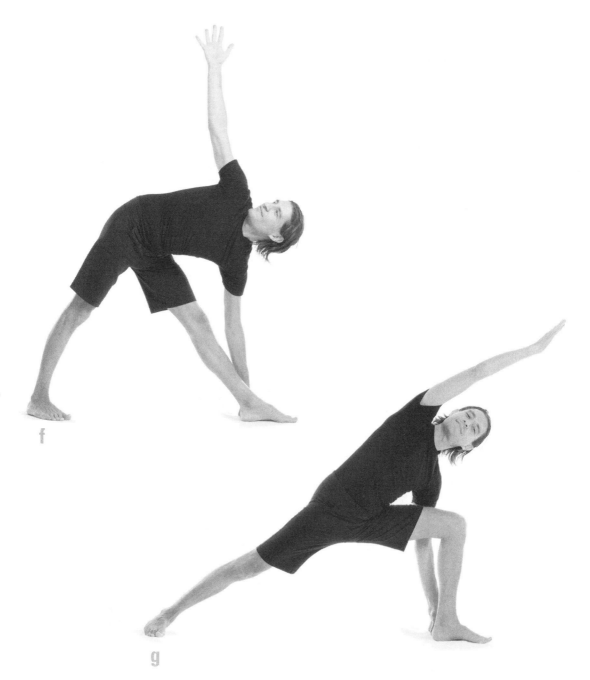

f

g

To come into parsva uttanasana, place the hands down to the floor at either side of the left foot. Inhale, lengthen the spine, and rotate the hips and shoulders forward. Then exhale, straighten the left leg into parsva uttanasana *(h)*, and stay for 6 breaths. To come into warrior III, bring the hands to the hips and bend the left leg slightly. Inhale and lift the right leg, keeping it parallel with the chest and keeping the right foot and the hips perpendicular to the floor. Exhale and straighten the left leg. Inhale, extending the arms in front of the body, and hold the warrior III pose *(i)* for 6 breaths. On the sixth inhalation lift to stand upright, taking the arms above the head as the right foot comes down to meet the left. Exhale and bring the palms together to the heart. Repeat the full vinyasa on the other side.

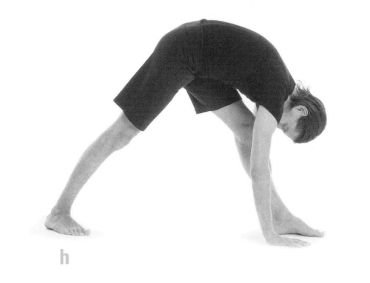

h

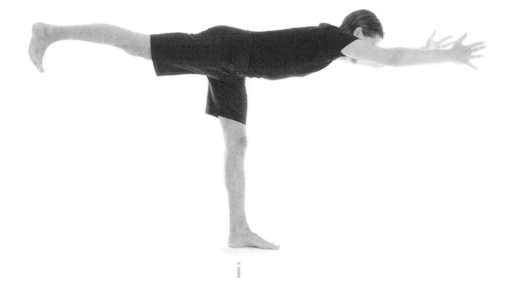

i

7. Triangle Twist (Parivrtti Trikonasana)

Stand in a wide split on the mat with the feet parallel. Inhale and reach the arms out to the sides (a). Exhale and twist, placing the left hand on the outside of the right foot as you extend the right arm up and gaze at the right hand. Inhale and lift back to center as you reach through both arms. Exhale and twist toward the left, placing the right hand to the outside of the left foot as you lift the left arm up and gaze at the left hand (b). Inhale, reaching through the arms, and lift back to center. Repeat the twist four times to each side, staying on the fourth repetition for 6 breaths on each side. Then inhale and lift back to center, reaching through both arms. Exhale and relax the arms to the sides.

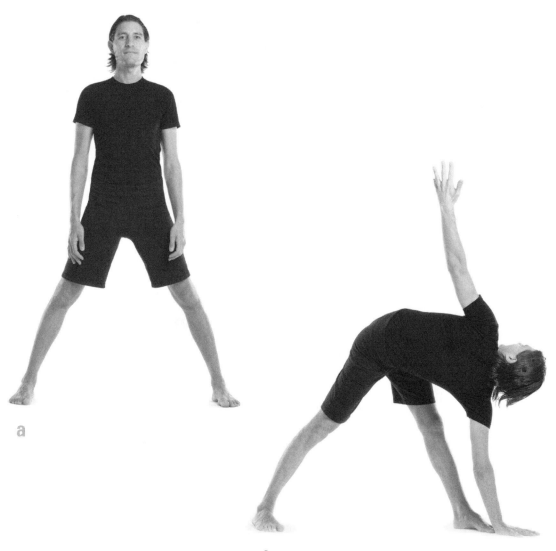

a

b

8. Tree (Vrksasana) to Extended Hand-to-Toe Pose (Utthita hasta padagusthasana) to Dancing Shiva (Natarajasana)

Stand at the front of the mat, gazing forward, with the feet together and the arms at the sides. Take the right hand to the right hip and place the left foot on the inside of the right thigh, with the knee out to the side. Extending upward through the right leg, fix your gaze on a point in front of the body and bring the palms together at the heart *(a)*. Inhale and lift the arms above the head with the palms together *(b)*. Stay in tree position for 5 breaths. On the fifth exhalation, relax the palms together back to the heart. Remain standing on the right leg, bring the left knee to the chest, and hold the left big toe with the first two fingers of the left hand. Inhale and come into utthita hasta padagusthasana by extending the left leg in front *(c)* of the body for 5 breaths.

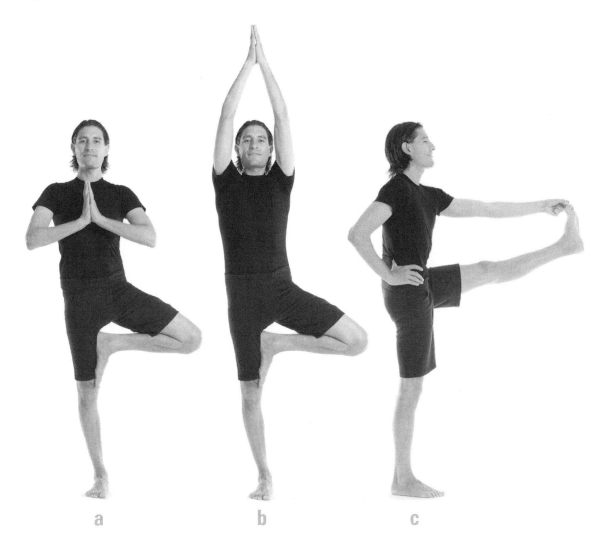

a   b   c

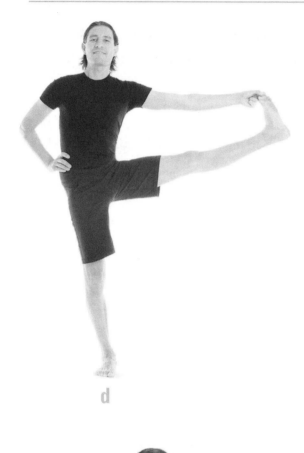

d

On the last inhalation open the left hip, taking the extended left leg out to the side *(d)*, and hold for 5 more breaths. On the last exhalation bring the extended left leg back in front of the body. Inhale and then exhale. Still holding the big toe, take the head toward the left knee *(e)* and hold for 5 more breaths. To come into natarajasana, or the dancing Shiva, inhale, lift the chest back up, release the big toe, and hold the inside of the left foot. Exhale, bend the left leg, and rotate the left shoulder to take the left leg behind the body *(f)*. Inhale and lift the right arm above the head, lifting through the chest for 5 more breaths. On the last exhalation release the left foot to the floor and relax the arms to the sides. Repeat the complete vinyasa on the other side.

e

f

9. One-Arm Balance (Vasisthasana) Vinyasa

Stand at the front of the mat with the feet together, the arms at the sides, and the gaze forward. Gazing up, inhale and lift the arms for the palms to meet above the head *(a)*. Start the exhalation and bend over the legs, bringing the hands to the floor at either side of the feet *(b)*. Inhale, lengthening the spine and lifting the chest. Exhale, deepening the forward bend and softening the knees. Hold the breath out and lightly hop back to a low push-up in chataranga dandasana, or stick pose, keeping the toes curled under *(c)*. Here the body should be lifted a few inches off the floor, with the elbows in close to the body and the shoulders back.

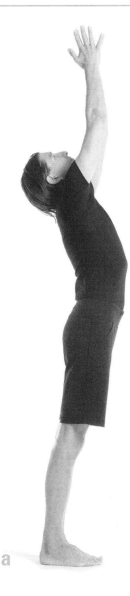

a

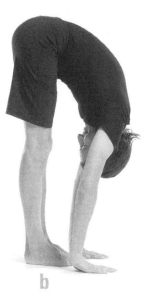

b

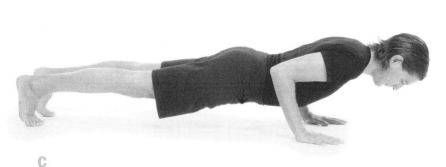

c

Intense 50- to 60-Minute Workout

Inhale, pivot forward to upward-facing dog *(d)*, and then exhale back to downward-facing dog *(e)* for 5 breaths. Keep the toes curled under, and inhale, pivoting forward to plank, with the arms straight and the body extending from the torso through the heels *(f)*. Then balance on the left hand, stacking the right foot on top of the left and placing the right hand on the right hip. Exhale and stabilize the base of the body through mula bandha. Then inhale and extend up the right arm, with the palm wide, into vasisthasana *(g)*. Look at the top hand and stay for 5 breaths.

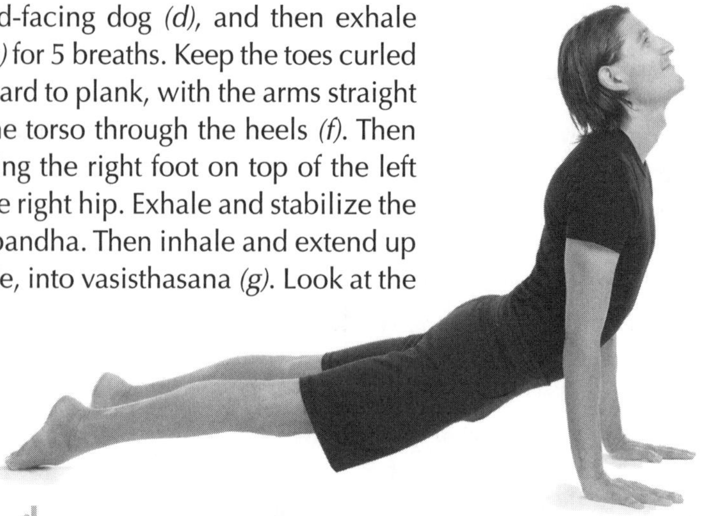

d

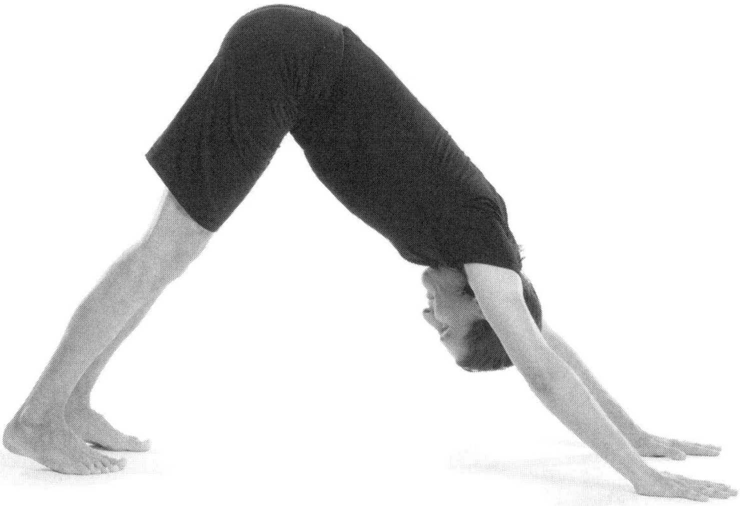

e

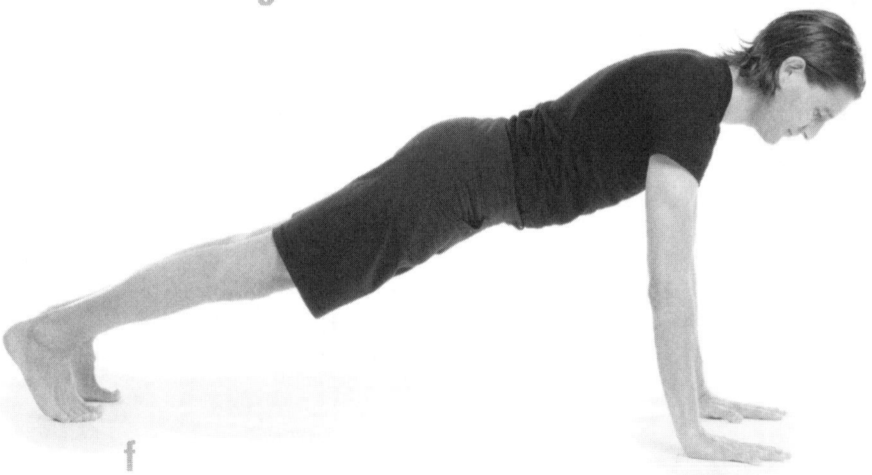

f

Then exhale, lower the right hand to the floor, and come back to plank pose *(f)*. Inhale to upward-facing dog *(d)* and exhale back to downward-facing dog *(e)*. Inhale and lower to hands and knees, lifting the chest and gazing up slightly, and exhale back to child's pose *(h)* for a moment of rest. Inhale and come back up to the hands and knees. Exhale back to downward-facing dog *(e)* again for 5 more breaths. Then inhale and pivot forward to plank pose *(f)*. Come back to vasisthasana *(g)*, this time balancing on the right hand with the left arm extended, for 5 breaths. Exhale and lower the left hand back to the floor into plank pose *(f)*. Inhale and then exhale, bending the elbows and lowering down to the floor.

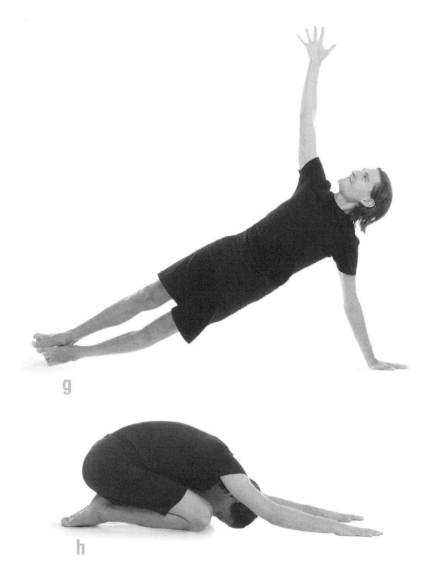

g

h

Intense 50- to 60-Minute Workout

10. Cobra (Bhujangasana) to Child's Pose (Balasana) to Standing on Knees

Lie face down, forehead on the floor and hands by the ribs, with the elbows facing up. Inhale and lift the head, neck, and chest into cobra *(a)*. Exhale and come back to child's pose *(b)* with the arms extended in front of the body. Inhale and stand on the knees, taking the arms overhead and lifting through the chest *(c)*. Exhale and lower back to child's pose, with the arms extended in front of the body. Inhale and slide through to a low cobra. Exhale and lower the forehead and chest to the floor. Repeat the sequence six times. Stay in cobra for 6 breaths on the last repetition and finish resting on the front of the body.

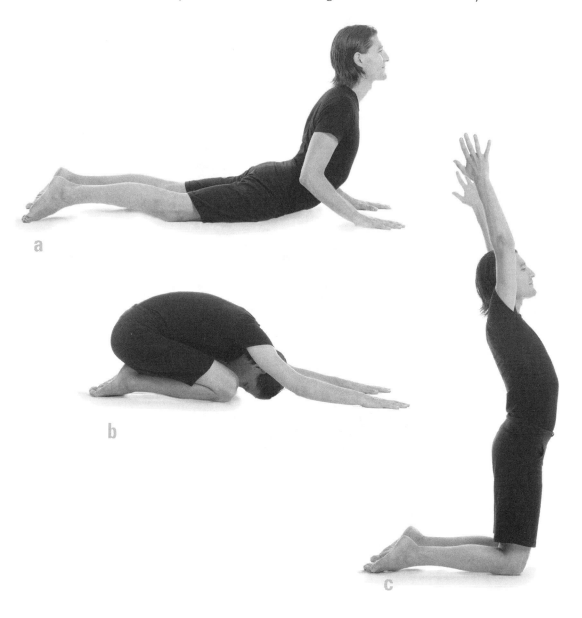

a

b

c

11. Bow (Dhanurasana)

Bend the legs and hold the ankles. Inhale, lifting the head, neck, chest, and legs, opening the heart, letting the shoulders roll back, and gazing up slightly. Stay in bow for 8 breaths, and then on the last exhalation lower down and release the feet. Bring the hands back by the ribs and come back to child's pose to rest.

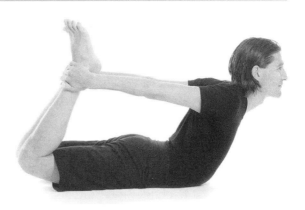

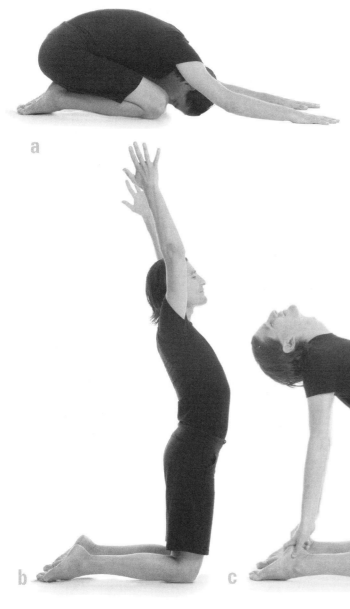

a

b

c

12. Camel (Ustrasana)

Start in child's pose with the arms extended in front of the body *(a)*. Inhale and lift up to stand on the knees, taking the arms overhead *(b)*. Remain standing on the knees and exhale, lowering the arms to hold the heels. Inhale, lift through the chest, and engage the legs to protect the lower back *(c)*. Exhale, relaxing the head back, and stay in camel for 6 breaths. Then inhale, release the heels, lift the head, and take the arms overhead. Exhale and come back down to child's pose and rest.

13. Headstand (Sirsasana)

Come up to the hands and knees and measure that the elbows are a forearm's width apart, and then interlace the fingers to form a cradle for the head. Place the back of the top of the head to the floor between the interlaced fingers. Curl the toes under, lift the hips, and walk the feet forward toward the elbows until the hips are lifted above the torso *(a)*. Balancing on the forearms and hands, with very little pressure on the head, bend the knees to the chest *(b)* and inhale, lifting the legs to stay in the headstand *(c)* for 12 breaths. Exhale and lower the legs straight to the floor. Bend the knees and release the head from the hands, then come back to child's pose and rest. Note that you can do both the headstand and the next pose, the forearm stand, by a wall for added support at first.

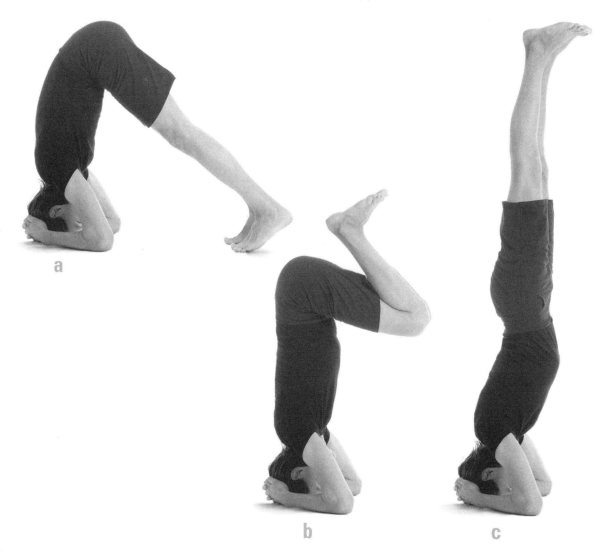

a

b

c

14. Forearm Stand (Pincha Mayurasana)

Lift up slightly from child's' pose and bring the palms, forearms, and elbows to the floor. Gazing forward, extend through the arms, straighten the legs, and walk the feet forward until the hips are lifted above the torso. Inhale and lift the right leg. Exhale, then inhale and lift the left leg as well, coming into the forearm stand. Hold for 12 breaths. Then exhale, lower the legs back down, and rest in child's pose.

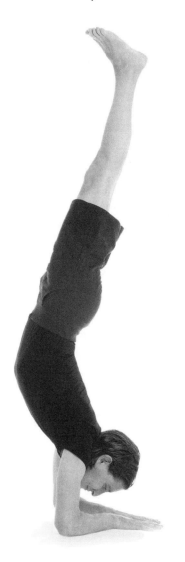

15. Shoulder Stand (Sarvangasana)

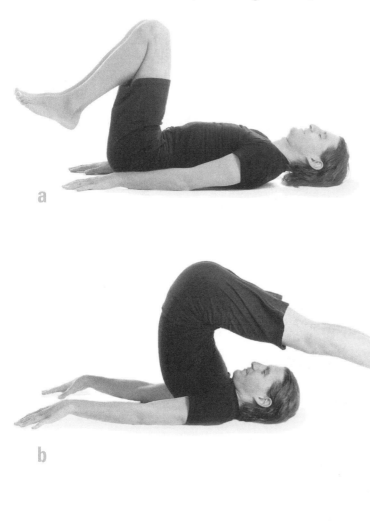

Lie on the back with the knees bent and the arms along the sides, palms facing down *(a)*. Inhale here, then exhale and roll onto the shoulders, bringing the feet to the floor behind the head *(b)*. Bend the elbows and place the hands on the back, with the palms flat and the elbows in comfortably close to the body. Inhale and lift the legs up to shoulder stand *(c)*. Stay for 12 breaths, engaging the front and back of the body by pointing through the feet and curling back just the toes.

16. Transition to One-Leg Bridge

From the shoulder stand, inhale and lower the right foot to the floor in front of the body, keeping the left leg lifted. Stay for 4 breaths. Then inhale and lower the left foot to the floor. Exhale, lift the right leg back up, and hold for 4 more breaths. Inhale and lower the right leg back down so that both feet are parallel on the mat. Stay for 4 breaths. Then release the palms from the back and exhale, lowering the hips to the floor.

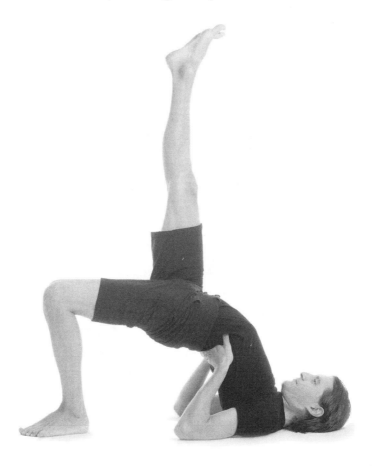

17. Wheel (Urdva Danurasana)

Start on the back with the feet parallel and at hip-width distance. Bring the palms by the ears with the fingers pointing toward the body *(a)*. Inhale here and then exhale, extending through the arms and legs and lifting directly into full wheel *(b)*. Stay for 8 breaths, grounding through the feet, opening through the chest, and relaxing the neck. On the last exhalation, tuck in the chin and lower down to the floor. Take a moment to rest and then do the wheel once more. Afterward hug in the knees to release the lower back.

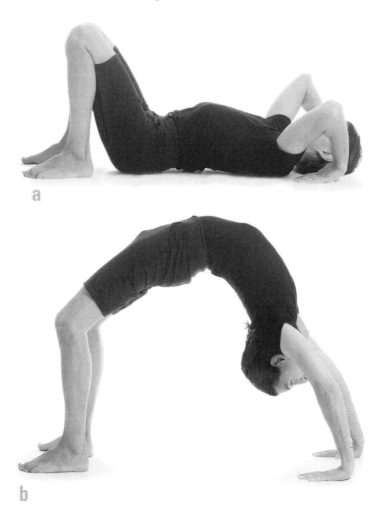

a

b

18. Fish Pose (Matsyasana)

Lying on the back, extend the legs long and take the arms under the body with the palms face down under the hips. Inhale and lift the torso, pressing through the elbows. Exhale and relax the top of the head to the floor, coming into a back arch. Hold the fish pose for 6 breaths, lifting through the chest, with very little pressure on the head itself. Then, staying in the back arch, on the last exhalation lift the legs off the floor and point through the feet.

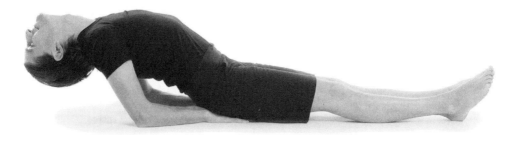

19. Boat (Navasana)

Coming from fish into boat pose with the legs lifted, inhale and lift the head, lowering the chin toward the chest and taking the hands out from under the body. Exhale and lift the arms, reaching beyond the extended legs. Stay in the boat pose for 6 breaths. Inhale, lower the legs to the floor, lift the torso upright to sitting, placing palms by the hips.

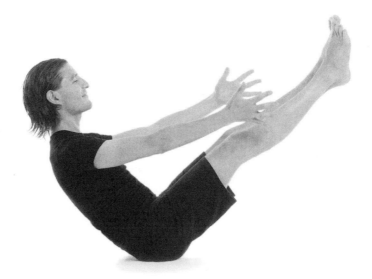

20. Seated Forward Bend (Pascimatanasana)

Sit upright with the legs long and the hands at either side of the hips. Inhale, bringing the arms overhead *(a)*. Exhale and bend over the legs, placing the hands over the feet *(b)*. Stay for 8 breaths. Inhale, lifting back up and taking the arms overhead. Exhale and relax the arms down.

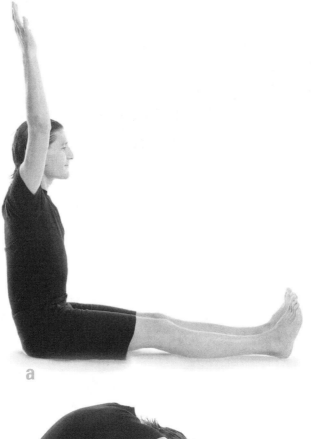

a

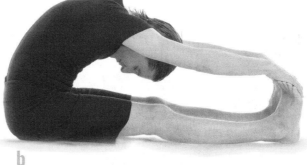

b

21. Seated Twist With Hand Gesture (Ardha Matsyendrasana With Mudra)

Place the right foot to the outside of the left thigh and then bend the left leg toward the body. Place the outer upper left arm to the outside of the right thigh and form a mudra (hand gesture) with the index finger and the thumb (see photo). Wrap the right arm around the body, placing the right hand to the inside of the left thigh. Turn the head toward the right and soften the gaze to bring the focus inward. Inhale, lengthening the spine, and exhale, deepening the twist and drawing the belly in and up, for 6 breaths. Then release the twist and repeat to the other side.

22. Ankle to Knee (Agnistambhasana)

Sitting upright, take the right leg in front of the body and bend the knee so that the right calf is extended facing the torso. Then take the left leg over the right, with the left foot over the outside of the right knee and the left knee in line with the right foot underneath it, forming a triangle between the legs and hips *(a)*. Place the hands to the floor in front of the body. Inhale, lifting through the chest, and then exhale, rounding the spine over the legs *(b)*. Stay in the pose for 6 breaths. Then inhale, lift the torso back up, release the legs, and switch legs to repeat the posture on the other side.

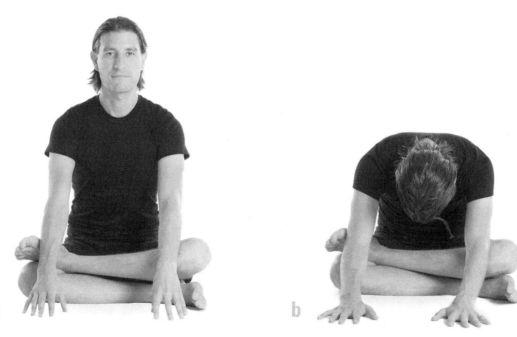

a

b

Intense 50- to 60-Minute Workout

23. Seated Ocean Breathing (Ujjayi Pranayama) With Bandha

Take a comfortable seated position with the arms extended, the palms on the knees facing up, and the chest lifting toward the chin. Close the eyes and form a chin mudra on both hands by touching the index finger and the thumb and extending the other fingers long. Inhale for 8 seconds using ocean breathing, and then lower the chin toward the chest to hold the breath in for 5 seconds. Keeping a long spine, exhale for 8 seconds, drawing the belly in and up. Lower the chin again, lift the chest, and hold the breath out for 5 seconds. Repeat this breath ratio for 4 breaths and then lengthen the next inhalation to 12 seconds. Hold the breath in for 8 seconds. Deepen the exhalation to 12 seconds. Now on the pause after the exhalation, lower the chin, lift the chest, and scoop the belly under the ribs to initiate udayana bandha and experience mula and jalandhara bandha together, for 8 seconds. Ease up and release the diaphragm, abdomen, and throat slightly prior to the next inhalation. Repeat this breathing technique and ratio for 10 more breaths. Then go back to the initial ratio of 8-second inhalation, 5-second pause, 8-second exhalation, 5-second pause for another 4 breaths. To finish the pranayama, breathe freely for a few moments and observe the breath coming and going with ease. Take a moment to fully experience your state of being prior to starting the rest of your day.

24. Hand-to-the-Heart Invocation

Sit in a cross-legged position with the palms together at the heart and the eyes closed. Inhale and lift the arms up the sides for the palms to meet overhead. Exhale and bring the palms together down to the heart. Repeat the breathing and movements three times to bring a heartfelt sense of openness and receptivity to the start of the day.

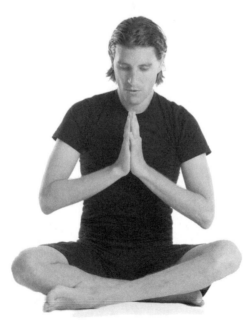

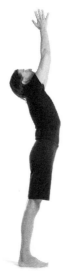

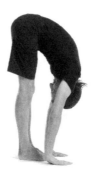

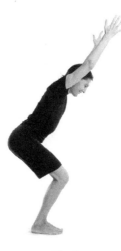

**Breathing Preparations
Mountain**

Standing Forward Bend

Chair

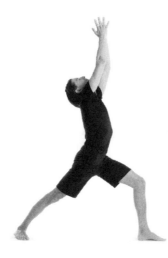

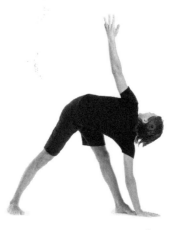

**Sun Salutation with Lunge
See pages 41-42**

**Warrior I Vinyasa
Repeat on the other side**

Triangle Twist

Intense 50- to 60-Minute Workout Guide

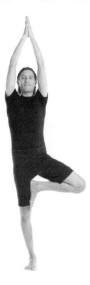

Tree Vinyasa
Repeat on the other side

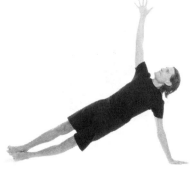

One-Arm Balance Vinyasa

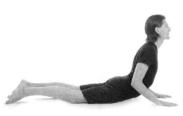

Cobra Vinyasa
Repeat 6 times

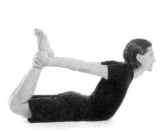

Bow

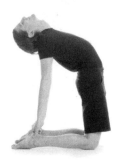

Camel

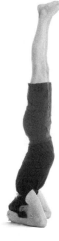

Headstand

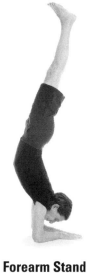

Forearm Stand

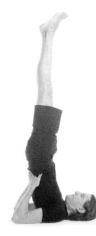

Shoulder Stand

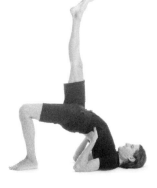

Transition to One-Leg Bridge

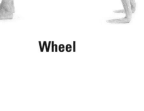

Wheel

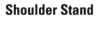
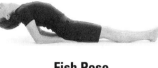

Fish Pose

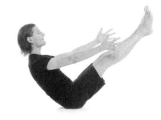

Boat

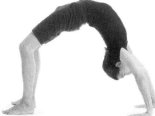

Seated Forward Bend

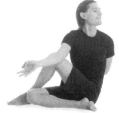

**Seated Twist
With Hand Gesture**

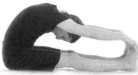

Ankle to Knee

**Seated Ocean Breathing
With Bandha
See page 200**

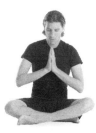

Hand-to-the-Heart Invocation

7

Visualization and Meditation

||||||||||||||||||||||||||||||||||||||||||||||||||||||||||||||||||||||||||||||||||||||||||||||||||||||||||||||||||||||||||||||||||||||||||||||||||||

The primary focus of the practices presented within this book has been asanas, vinyasas, and simple pranayamas, the latter being specific breathing exercises at the end of the practices to calm and focus the mind. I find these tools to be the most accessible and useful to the most people on a regular basis. However, the yoga tradition is as rich and diverse as it is old. So many practices, tools, and methods are associated with yoga tradition, all of which are intended to help individuals realize their full potential by living useful, healthy, and fulfilling lives. In addition to describing the physical postures and breathing exercises that compose the majority of our morning yoga workouts, I'd like to present the use of *mantra* (sound), *yantra* (yogic geometry), and creative visualization and simple observation of experience as means of going deeper, to a more subtle level of mindful self-awareness.

When we use sound and visualization, yoga can reflect our own creative personal expression and allows us to realize our inner vision. I don't consider these practices to be religious or contradictory to any personal beliefs, whatever they may be. Mantras (seed sounds), yantra, (yogic geometry), and meditative visualization can help anyone connect more fully to their inherent nature and to integrate the spirit of these practices with any religious or philosophical ideas that they believe in.

Mantras and Sound

Let's first discuss the use of simple mantras within asanas, pranayamas, and meditation. These mantras are in Sanskrit, an ancient scholarly language of India, in which all of the ancient teachings of yoga were originally handed down verbally from teacher to student for generations, prior to the existence of the first written text on yoga. The ancient yogis, through their meditative practices, constructed the language so that each syllable and root sound, or *bija mantra*, contained what they believed to be the essence of the universe. These mantras have certain vibrational effects that, when chanted, are both pleasant and powerful in their effect on the body, mind, and spirit. When chanting mantras you can easily clear the mind, because the chanting itself is such a concentrated activity. Chanting mantras during the asana practice, either with the movements or afterward as an adjunct practice, results in a clear mind and a sense of openness. There are many mantras—they really constitute an entire branch of yoga all by themselves. So we will only concentrate on a few that are relevant to our morning yoga.

The foremost root mantra is *Om*, pronounced "aum." It is represented by the symbol in figure 7.1, which many of us have become familiar with. The mantra Om represents the infinite entirety of the universe—the beginning, middle, and end of all things. With this simple mantra we acknowledge our connection to and our place within the incomprehensible vastness of the universe. The ancient yogis believed that by chanting "Om," one could unblock any obstacle that hindered a complete experience of our infinite nature.

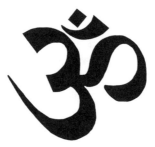

FIGURE 7.1 Symbol for *Om.*
Reprinted, by permission, from M. Kirk and B. Boon, 2004, *Hatha yoga illustrated* (Champaign, IL: Human Kinetics), 23.

Another mantra that we'll use is *Sohum*, pronounced "so-hum," which translates to "I am that." Together with Om it means "I am that that is everything" or "I am one with the universe." Let's try a simple exercise with movements to see how we can use these two together in a practice.

1. Come to a cross-legged seated position with the chest lifted and the palms together at the heart, and inhale.
2. Chanting "Om," take the arms up the sides for the palms to meet above the head. Gaze up slightly and then inhale.

3. Start to chant "Sohum," and take the palms together to the heart, lowering the chin toward the chest.

4. Repeat the chanting and movements three times and then rest with the palms at the heart.

5. Then relax the hands down to the knees, turn the palms to face up, and touch the index fingers to the thumbs. Close the eyes and take 6 more breaths, chanting "Om," silently in your mind as you inhale and then "Sohum" silently as you exhale.

To invoke the qualities of the sun we'll use the mantra *Surya,* pronounced "soor-ya," which in Sanskrit means the sun. This is a nice addition as we are doing yoga in the morning, a time of day when linking ourselves consciously to the life-giving energy and warmth of the sun is particularly powerful. Try the same exercise we just did, but this time use the mantra Surya in place of Sohum. Chant "Om Surya," meaning, "I am everything that is the sun," or "I realize the nature of the sun within myself."

Several other bija mantras constitute a verbal sun salutation, or surya namascar. Each one is composed of part of the Sanskrit vowel chain and represents a different aspect of the color spectrum that the light of the sun provides. These mantras are *Hram, Hrim, Hrum, Hraim, Hraum,* and *Hraha.* You can link these mantras with specific movements within the kneeling sun salutation, chanting one mantra on each movement and breathing in between. Let's try doing the exercises while chanting these bija mantras.

1. Place a blanket at the center of the mat and come to the hands and knees. Inhale, looking up and lifting the chest.

2. Chanting "Hram," pivot the hips forward to a moderate upward-facing dog and then inhale.

3. Chanting "Hrim," curl the toes under and lift the hips to downward-facing dog. Inhale.

4. Chanting "Hrum," lower back down to the hands and knees, looking up and lifting the chest. Inhale.

5. Chanting "Hraim," lower the hips to the heels and the forehead to the floor in child's pose, and then inhale.

6. Chanting "Hraum," lift all the way up to stand on the knees, taking the arms overhead, and then inhale standing on the knees.

7. Chanting "Hraha," lower back down to child's pose.

8. Inhale and lift back up to the hands and knees to start the sequence again. Then repeat the chanting and movements six more times.

The last mantra that I'd like to offer for your use is *Shanti,* meaning peace. I believe inner peace and a sense of freedom is the highest aim in yoga. If we can bring these qualities into ourselves through practice, using some of the tools and practices outlined in this book, then perhaps we are doing our part to increase peace with others and, as a result, elevate the level of peace in our society as a whole. Positive transformation starts with each one of us expanding our consciousness through self-developing activities like yoga. After your yoga asanas and pranayamas, try just chanting "Om Shanti" three times, either silently or aloud, to bring both the intention and awareness of peace into your day before getting up from the yoga mat.

Yantras and Visualizations

To create an awareness of the relationship between our physical form and our experience of the energetic currents within and around us, we can use the realm of inner vision, color, and light to creatively add an additional dimension to yoga and meditation. Visualization of color, light, and shape into our consciousness has a beneficial energetic effect on our senses. Specific shapes, traditionally known in the Vedic arts as yantras, are literally meant to map out how energy manifests itself in nature and within our systems. The simplest and yet most useful yantra is the intersection of equilateral triangles representing the balance of polarities, both in ourselves and in nature as a whole. The upward-pointing triangle represents *Shiva*, or masculine energy. The downward-pointing energy represents *Shakti*, or the feminine earth energy (see figure 7.2).

The practice of asana and pranayama in hatha yoga is meant to be a conscious participation in, and balancing of, the interplay of these two energies within our own system. The Shiva energy is penetrating, stabilizing, and grounding, whereas the Shakti energy, equally strong, is animated, free-flowing, and expansive. Shiva energy needs to be countered by Shakti to prevent its inherent rigidity and controlling tendencies. Likewise Shakti must be balanced by Shiva, because it can be uncontrollably powerful and potentially destructive, like a hurricane, when unfocused. Together Shiva and Shakti dance with each other in perfect union and balance, and for this reason the yantra is the perfect intersection of two equilateral triangles. At the center of the two triangles, where the two energies are in perfect equanimity and balance, is the *bindu*. Here we will place the visualization of color. For morning yoga, the color of that bindu should be bright orange or yellow, like the light of the sun. Let's try a simple meditation using the yantra.

1. Come to a comfortable cross-legged position with the hands at the knees, the spine straight, the arms long, the palms facing up, and the index fingers touching the thumbs.
2. Close the eyes and bring the focus inward.
3. Visualize a perfect circle encompassing a vertical perimeter around your entire self, from the head to the toes.
4. Now envision within the circle a triangle pointing downward to represent the Shakti or feminine earth energy. Take 4 steady long ujjayi breaths, visualizing the downward triangle in conjunction with the lengthy inhalation.
5. Now add to the visualization within the circle an upward-pointing triangle that perfectly intersects the first triangle. Continue with 4 more ujjayi breaths,

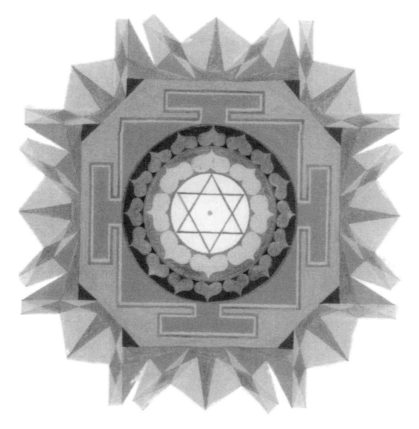

FIGURE 7.2   Triangles representing Shiva and Shakti.
Illustrated by Melissa Forbes.

this time visualizing the downward-facing triangle in conjunction with the strength of the exhalation, which is initiated by drawing the lower abdomen in and up.

6. Now visualize both triangles perfectly balanced within the circle surrounding you, giving each equal emphasis and concentration during the ujjayi inhalations and exhalations, for 4 more breaths.

7. Release the breath and continue to visualize and meditate on the two triangles within the circle that encompasses the perimeter of your physical being. Add the additional element of the bindu at the center of the circle and triangles, right at the center of the chest or heart region. Now visualize that point being bright yellow or orange and expansive, like the sun. Continue to sit this way for several minutes, visualizing the sun's energy at the heart region, the bindu at the center of the circle, the perfect point of balance between the two triangles that form the yantra.

8. When you feel ready, release the visualization and place the heels of the palms to the eyes. With the heels of the palms pressed ever so slightly, relax the face and bring your awareness to it, noticing any colors or shapes that lie in the inner vision behind the eyelids.

9. Stay for a few moments, observing and enjoying the play of color and shape within your inner vision, freely and without effort.

10. Then relax the hands down and open your eyes.

The simple practices that use both sound and visualization offer a creative depth to the practices outlined in the book. Feel free to play with them, without a sense of imposition or necessity. The real magic of the yoga is the sheer enjoyment of doing it and the many benefits that your intentions and efforts produce.

Breath Observation Meditation

Perhaps the most challenging and rewarding practice we can add to our yoga is the simple meditation of observing the breath. In this practice we just sit quietly in a comfortable position—cross-legged; kneeling using blankets, blocks, or a cushion; or even in a chair if necessary to maintain comfort and stillness for some time. Once we have ourselves situated in a seated posture with the spine long and the hands cupped facing up in the lap or grounded on our knees, we relax the face and let go of any methods of breathing we have used earlier in practice. Sitting with the eyes closed or gazing softly ahead, we bring awareness to areas of tension within our bodies and allow them to soften through simple acknowledgment. Then we bring our thoughts to the natural occurrence of the breath, focusing on each exhalation as it occurs, and letting go even further as we receive the inhalation freely. Continue to sit and observe for just a few moments, at first gently noticing the mind's tendency to run off in various directions with the thoughts that move through our consciousness. Playfully bring the awareness back to the breath. At first try this for just a minute or so, and through continued practice notice your natural tendency to sit slightly longer, with more enjoyment. Doing this observing meditation can truly allow us to relax and fully energize our spirits through an open connection to the simplicity of the present moment.

Tying It All Together

Meditations of sound, vision, and the profoundly simple observation of breath infuse a fulfilling layer of spiritual depth and meaning to our morning yoga work-out. Being mindful of breath and body and using sound and vision to evoke the nuances of the mind can help us cultivate a peaceful sense of empowerment, enabling us to develop compassion for others and ourselves. Through regular practice we may come to realize that the health of our bodies is truly interrelated with the nature of our thoughts and with our capacity to breathe smoothly through the many challenges of life. Starting our days with the active meditation of body, breath, mind, and spirit as a morning yoga workout will positively transform our lives and benefit others in beautiful and unforeseen ways.

Index of Yoga Asanas

Seated Asanas

Standing Asanas

Prone Asanas

Supine Asanas

Arm-Supported Asanas

Kneeling Asanas

Inverted Asanas

Index

Note: The italicized *f* following pages numbers refers to figures.

About the Author

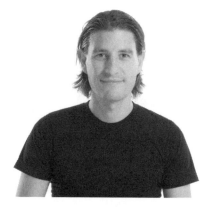

Zack Kurland is a yoga therapist in New York City, where he lives with his wife and son. He is a member of the teaching staff at OM yoga center, where he trains teachers in yoga therapy; is certified through the Heart of Yoga Association; and is a member of the Yoga Alliance and the International Association of Yoga Therapists. Kurland continues to educate himself in yoga therapy and Ayurveda in the United States and India. He has written articles for and been featured in *Fit Yoga* magazine and *Yoga Journal*.

For more information on Zack Kurland yoga therapy, upcoming workshops, and yoga therapy trainings, visit www.zackkurland.com.

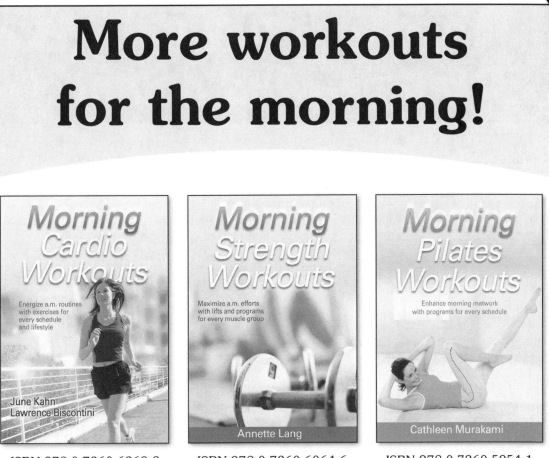

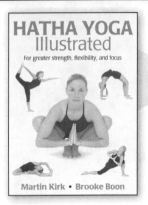
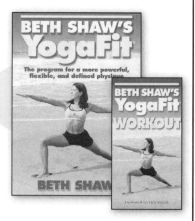
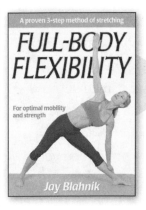